THE EMPAYS

"A virtuosic manifesto of human pain. . . . Jamison stitches together
the intellectual and the emotional with the finesse of a crackerjack
surgeon. . . . The result is a soaring performance on the humanizing
effects of empathy."   —National Public Radio

"[A] stunning collection. . . . A profound investigation of empathy's
potential and its limits."
                      —*Cosmopolitan*, "10 Books by Women You Have to
                                         Read This Spring"

"If reading a book about [pain] sounds . . . painful, rest assured that
Jamison writes with such originality and humor, and delivers such
scalpel-sharp insights, that it's more like a rush of pleasure. . . . To
articulate suffering with so much clarity, and so little judgment, is
to turn pain into art."   —*Entertainment Weekly*

"Jamison writes with sober precision and unusual vulnerability,
with a tendency to circle back and reexamine, to deconstruct and
anticipate the limits of her own perspective, and a willingness to
make her own medical and psychological history the objects of her
examinations. Her insights are often piercing and poetic."
                      —*The New Yorker*'s "Page-Turner,"
                                        "Books to Watch Out For"

"Even before rave reviews propelled Leslie Jamison's essay collection onto best-seller lists, I found myself doing some math as I read her remarkable book, which deserves as big an audience as it can get. At thirty, she could be a granddaughter of Joan Didion and Susan Sontag, whose nonfiction debuts first stirred up readers nearly half a century ago. They set a daunting standard for the power of alert nerves, in *Slouching Towards Bethlehem*, and of fierce thoughts, in *Against Interpretation*. *The Empathy Exams* is their descendant, yet Jamison's blend of wit and brainy warmth is completely distinctive."
—*The Atlantic*

"[An] excellent new collection. . . . The question at its core is what we humans should do about suffering, and Jamison reframes it again and again, in settings from the border crossing at Tijuana to a murder trial to the finish line of an ultramarathon."   —*New York*

"If this first essay collection is a predictor, then Leslie Jamison may just be the next great American lady of letters."
—GQ, "8 Books You Need to Read This April"

"[A] thoughtful collection of essays interrogating the physical and metaphorical meanings of pain. . . . Jamison is compassionate without being partial."   —*The New Yorker*

"Poetic, painfully searching essays about violence, sex, illness, self-esteem and self-expression."   —*Associated Press*

"A brilliant collection. . . . We're in a new golden age of the essay . . . and in *The Empathy Exams* Leslie Jamison has announced herself as its rising star."   —*The Boston Globe*

"Remarkable. . . . [Jamison] combines the intellectual rigor of a philosopher, the imagination of a novelist and a reporter's keen eye for detail in these essays, which seamlessly blend reportage, cultural criticism, theory, and memoir."   —*Los Angeles Times*

"A lush, erudite collection. . . . One could say about Jamison, as she says here about Joan Didion, 'Her intelligence excavates a truth at once uncomfortable and crystalline.'" —*The Washington Post*

"[Jamison] writes with intellectual precision and a deep emotional engagement. . . . *The Empathy Exams* is a gracefully powerful attempt by a tremendously talented young writer to articulate the ways in which we might all work to become better versions of ourselves." —*Star Tribune* (Minneapolis)

"A striking collection of essays. . . . [Jamison's] self-awareness may be the collection's greatest strength, allowing Jamison to lay bare the insecurities and insufficiencies in how she—and by extension we—practice empathy." —*The Kansas City Star*

"Deeply thoughtful." —*Chicago Tribune*

"As a study in vulnerability, but also in types of speech and silence that surround the ailing body, *The Empathy Exams* is exceptional, Jamison concluding that empathy is a matter of the hardest work, 'made of exertion, that dowdier cousin of impulse.'" —*The Guardian* (UK)

"If this is the new age of the essay, Jamison is one of the form's most compelling voices. *The Empathy Exams* is a challenging book, pushing the reader forward even when the subject matter grows gruesome or difficult. It gives us a map, drawn in fits and starts, for navigating human interaction." —*New Statesman* (UK)

"These essays walk a knife-edge between self and social inquiry. . . . Pace yourself when you read this short, visceral book, let each essay resound before moving on to another." —*The Independent* (UK)

"Jamison is in total command of her material, able to swing from dry precision to poetry. But it is her ability to notice and needle her own artifice that makes her work fly. Her gaze is sharp and turns inward as often as outward." —*Financial Times* (UK)

"Based on this book, Leslie Jamison is very much the next thing in nonfiction. A writer of uncommon intelligence, she merges memoir with reportage and criticism to create something not entirely new, but certainly novel and definitely exciting."   —*Maclean's* (Canada)

"[Jamison] circles around questions without settling for easy answers."   —*The Columbus Dispatch*

"Fiercely contemplative, confessional essays. . . . [An] intelligent book."   —*The Plain Dealer* (Cleveland)

"Stunning. . . . A brutally honest, sometimes funny, always touching portrait of a woman growing up and moving through a complicated world."   —*The Gazette* (Cedar Rapids)

"Brilliant. . . . Jamison offers no all-purpose definition of empathy. That is, perhaps, her greatest contribution to the conversation: she invites us to think harder about what empathy might be—to excavate its layers—to approach empathy with more empathy, yes."
—*Los Angeles Review of Books*

"Jamison is determined to tell us what she sees and thinks without condescension or compromise, and as a consequence her act of witnessing is moving, stimulating, and disturbing in equal measure. . . . Jamison is always interesting, often gripping."   —*Bookforum*

"Revelatory. . . . [Jamison] proves herself at once unreliable and commanding, showing us her own queasiness in a way that can only inspire our confidence. And, of course, our empathy."
—*The American Scholar*

"Extraordinary. . . . Much of the intellectual charge of Jamison's writing comes from the sense that she is always looking for ways to examine her own reactions to things; no sooner has she come to some judgment or insight than she begins searching for a way to overturn it, or to deepen its complications. She flinches, and then she explores that flinch with a steady gaze. . . . [A] beautiful and punishing book."   —*Slate*

"An extraordinary essay collection driven by a fierce, piercing intelligence laced with endless amounts of curiosity about the world and the thoughts, feelings, and ability that make us humans. . . . It's a startling work of nonfiction that deserves every accolade it's going to receive, and it announces a voice that you'll want to follow anywhere." —*Flavorwire*

"While Jamison refreshingly offers no clear-cut answers or solutions, she does offer hope—for what we owe each other, for what we may be capable of giving. *The Empathy Exams* is essay at its finest—transformative, and here just in time." —*The Daily Beast*

"Stunning. . . . The range of *The Empathy Exams* recalls John Jeremiah Sullivan; Jamison's vulnerability evokes a less sentimental Cheryl Strayed." —*Grantland*

"[Jamison makes] sharp observations about how people respond to pain and how people respond to other people's pain. In *The Empathy Exams*, Jamison's essays do a rare thing: they show us—in many ways—what empathy means." —*The Millions*

"Jamison contemplates what it is to feel, how we communicate what we feel and what we do with these communications. . . . Readers will finish with no doubt she is sincere in her quest to own, identify and comprehend empathy." —*Shelf Awareness*

"This book melted my brain and my heart several times. . . . Jamison is at once journalistic and intimate, and there were moments in 'Grand Unified Theory of Female Pain' that actually made me feel like my heart would overflow with the kinship I felt to her." —*Book Riot*

"Jamison's exploration of the upsides, downsides, and difficulties of empathy is insightful, thought provoking, and itself empathetic. . . . A must read." —*Bustle*

"If empathy is setting our own discomfort to allow the feelings or symptoms of others to become our feelings, too, than entering into an empathetic contract with Jamison is a worthwhile exercise. These are essays that challenge and provoke, affirm and affect." —*Bookslut*

"Reading Leslie Jamison for the first time, you feel like you have been let in on a great secret. . . . Jamison's *The Empathy Exams* grants the sense that she has all of the goods to be one of the great commentators of our time. She has a keen eye for observation, an exceptional gift for a turn of phrase, and an adventurous spirit."
—*Washington Independent Review of Books*

"[Jamison] manages—with a novelist's eye for detail and scene setting—to come across as a Montaignian figure, full of doubt, heart, and a yearning to expand the boundaries of the fragile self."
—*Tin House*

"A heady and unsparing examination of pain and how it allows us to understand others, and ourselves. . . . Jamison is ever-probing and always sensitive. Reporting is never the point; instead, her observations of people, reality TV, music, film, and literature serve as a starting point for unconventional metaphysical inquiries into poverty, tourism, prison time, random acts of violence, abortion, HBO's *Girls*, bad romance, and stereotypes of the damaged woman artist." —*Publishers Weekly*, starred review, "Pick of the Week"

"A dazzling collection of essays on the human condition. . . . Jamison exhibits at once a journalist's courage to bear witness to acts and conditions that test human limits . . . and a poet's skepticism at her own motives for doing so. It is this level of scrutiny that lends these provocative explorations both earthy authenticity and moving urgency. A fierce, razor-sharp, heartwarming nonfiction debut."
—*Kirkus Reviews*, starred review

"Jamison examines some very difficult topics with intelligent candor. . . . These essays will inspire readers to reflect on their own feelings of empathy—not an easy feat in today's disinterested society."
—*Library Journal*, starred review

"Gutsy essays. . . . A tough, intrepid, scouring observer and vigilant thinker, [Jamison] generates startling and sparkling extrapolations and analysis. On the prowl for truth and intimate with pain, Jamison carries forward the fierce and empathic tradition as practiced by writers she names as mentors, most resonantly James Agee and Joan Didion."
—*Booklist*, starred review

"Leslie Jamison has written a profound exploration into how empathy deepens us, yet how we unwittingly sabotage our own capacities for it. We care because we are porous, she says. Pain is at once actual and constructed, feelings are made based on how you speak them. This riveting book will make you a better writer, a better human."
—Mary Karr, author of *Lit* and *The Liar's Club*

"*The Empathy Exams* is a book without an anaesthetic, a work of tremendous pleasure and tremendous pain. Leslie Jamison is alternately surgeon, midwife, psychiatrist, radiologist, and nurse—and in all these things she is fiercely intelligent, fiercely compassionate, and fiercely, prodigiously brave. This is the essay at its creative, philosophical best."
—Eleanor Catton, author of *The Luminaries*, winner of the Man Booker Prize

"These essays—risky, brilliant, and full of heart—ricochet between what it is to be alive and to be a creature wondering what it is to be alive. Jamison's words, torqued to a perfect balance, shine brightly, allowing both fury and wonder to open inside us."
—Nick Flynn, author of *Another Bullshit Night in Suck City*

"*The Empathy Exams* is a necessary book, a brilliant antidote to the noise of our time. . . . It earns its place on the shelf alongside Susan Sontag's *Regarding the Pain of Others* and *Illness as Metaphor* and Virginia Woolf's odd but stunning essay, 'On Being Ill.'"
—Charles D'Ambrosio, author of *The Dead Fish Museum* and *Loitering: New and Collected Essays*

"In *The Empathy Exams*, Leslie Jamison positions herself in one fraught subject position after the next: tourist in the suffering of others, guilt-ridden person of privilege, keenly intelligent observer distrustful of pure cleverness, reclaimer and critic of female suffering, to name but a few. She does so in order to probe her endlessly important and difficult subject—empathy, for the self and for others—a subject this whirling collection of essays turns over rock after rock to explore. Its perambulations are wide-ranging; its attentiveness to self and others, careful and searching; its open heart, true."
—Maggie Nelson, author of *The Art of Cruelty: A Reckoning* and *Bluets*

"Leslie Jamison threads her fine mind through the needle of emotion, sewing our desire for feeling to our fear of feeling. Her essays pierce both pain and sweetness."
—Eula Biss, author of *On Immunity: An Inoculation* and *Notes from No Man's Land: American Essays*

"Leslie Jamison writes with her whole heart and an unconfined intelligence, a combination that gives *The Empathy Exams*—an inquiry into modern ways and problems of feeling—a persuasive, often thrilling authority. These essays reach out for the world, seeking the extraordinary, the bizarre, the alone, the unfeeling, and finding always what is human."
—Michelle Orange, author of *This Is Running for Your Life*

"Brilliant. At times steel-cold or chili-hot, [Jamison] picks her way through a society that has lost its way, a voyeur of voyeurism. Here now comes the post-Sontag, post-modern American essay."
—Ed Vulliamy, author of *Amexica: War along the Borderline*

THE
EMPATHY EXAMS

Also by Leslie Jamison

The Gin Closet

The Empathy Exams

‡ ESSAYS ‡

Leslie Jamison

GRAYWOLF PRESS

This publication is made possible, in part, by the voters of Minnesota through a Minnesota State Arts Board Operating Support grant, thanks to a legislative appropriation from the arts and cultural heritage fund, and through grants from the National Endowment for the Arts and the Wells Fargo Foundation Minnesota. Significant support has also been provided by Target, the McKnight Foundation, Amazon.com, and other generous contributions from foundations, corporations, and individuals. To these organizations and individuals we offer our heartfelt thanks.

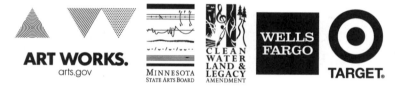

Published by Graywolf Press
250 Third Avenue North, Suite 600
Minneapolis, Minnesota 55401

All rights reserved.

www.graywolfpress.org

Published in the United States of America

ISBN 978-1-55597-671-2

12 14 16 15 13 11

Library of Congress Control Number: 2013946927

Cover design: Kimberly Glyder Design

For my mother,

Joanne Leslie

Homo sum: humani nil a me alienum puto

I am human: nothing human is alien to me.

—TERENCE, *The Self-Tormentor*

Contents

THE
⁑ EMPATHY EXAMS ⁑

My job title is medical actor, which means I play sick. I get paid by the hour. Medical students guess my maladies. I'm called a standardized patient, which means I act toward the norms set for my disorders. I'm standardized-lingo SP for short. I'm fluent in the symptoms of preeclampsia and asthma and appendicitis. I play a mom whose baby has blue lips.

Medical acting works like this: You get a script and a paper gown. You get $13.50 an hour. Our scripts are ten to twelve pages long. They outline what's wrong with us—not just what hurts but how to express it. They tell us how much to give away, and when. We are supposed to unfurl the answers according to specific protocol. The scripts dig deep into our fictive lives: the ages of our children and the diseases of our parents, the names of our husbands' real estate and graphic design firms, the amount of weight we've lost in the past year, the amount of alcohol we drink each week.

My specialty case is Stephanie Phillips, a twenty-three-year-old who suffers from something called conversion disorder. She is grieving the death of her brother, and her grief has sublimated into seizures. Her disorder is news to me. I didn't know you could convulse from sadness. She's not supposed to know, either. She's not supposed to think the seizures have anything to do with what she's lost.

STEPHANIE PHILLIPS
Psychiatry
SP Training Materials

CASE SUMMARY: You are a twenty-three-year-old female patient experiencing seizures with no identifiable neurological origin. You can't remember your seizures but are told you froth at the mouth and yell obscenities. You can usually feel a seizure coming before it arrives. The seizures began two years ago, shortly after your older brother drowned in the river just south of the Bennington Avenue Bridge. He was swimming drunk after a football tailgate. You and he worked at the same miniature-golf course. These days you don't work at all. These days you don't do much. You're afraid of having a seizure in public. No doctor has been able to help you. Your brother's name was Will.

MEDICATION HISTORY: You are not taking any medications. You've never taken antidepressants. You've never thought you needed them.

MEDICAL HISTORY: Your health has never caused you any trouble. You've never had anything worse than a broken arm. Will was there when you broke it. He was the one who called the paramedics and kept you calm until they came.

Our simulated exams take place in three suites of purpose-built rooms. Each room is fitted with an examination table and a surveillance camera. We test second- and third-year medical students in topical rotations: pediatrics, surgery, psychiatry. On any given exam day, each student must go through "encounters"—their technical title—with three or four actors playing different cases.

A student might have to palpate a woman's ten-on-scale-of-ten abdominal pain, then sit across from a delusional young lawyer and tell him that when he feels a writhing mass of worms in his small intestine, the feeling is probably coming from somewhere else. Then this med student might arrive in my room, stay straight faced, and tell me that I'm about to go into premature labor to deliver the pillow strapped to my belly, or nod solemnly as I express concern about my ailing plastic baby: "He's just so quiet."

Once the fifteen-minute encounter has ended, the medical student leaves the room, and I fill out an evaluation of his/her performance. The first part is a checklist: Which crucial pieces of information did he/she manage to elicit? Which ones did he/she leave uncovered? The second part of the evaluation covers affect.

Checklist item 31 is generally acknowledged as the most important category: "Voiced empathy for my situation/problem." We are instructed about the importance of this first word, *voiced*. It's not enough for someone to have a sympathetic manner or use a caring tone. The students have to say the right words to get credit for compassion.

We SPs are given our own suite for preparation and decompression. We gather in clusters: old men in crinkling blue robes, MFAs in boots too cool for our paper gowns, local teenagers in hospital ponchos and sweatpants. We help each other strap pillows around our waists. We hand off infant dolls. Little pneumonic Baby Doug, swaddled in a cheap cotton blanket, is passed from girl to girl like a relay baton. Our ranks are full of community-theater actors and undergrad drama majors seeking stages, high school kids earning booze money, retired folks with spare time. I am a writer, which means I'm trying not to be broke.

We play a demographic menagerie: Young jocks with ACL injuries and business executives nursing coke habits. STD Grandma has just cheated on her husband of forty years and has a case of gonorrhea to show for it. She hides behind her shame like a veil, and her med student is supposed to part the curtain. If he asks the right questions, she'll have a simulated crying breakdown halfway through the encounter.

Blackout Buddy gets makeup: a gash on his chin, a black eye, and bruises smudged in green eye shadow along his cheekbone. He's been in a fender bender he can't even remember. Before the encounter, the actor splashes booze on his body like cologne. He's supposed to let the particulars of his alcoholism glimmer through, very "unplanned," bits of a secret he's done his best to keep guarded.

Our scripts are studded with moments of flourish: Pregnant Lila's husband is a yacht captain sailing overseas off Croatia. Appendicitis Angela has a dead guitarist uncle whose tour bus was hit by a tornado. Many of our extended family members have died violent midwestern deaths: mauled in tractor or grain-elevator accidents, hit by drunk drivers on the way home from Hy-Vee grocery stores, felled

by big weather or Big-Ten tailgates (firearm accident)—or, like my
brother Will, by the quieter aftermath of debauchery.

Between encounters, we are given water, fruit, granola bars, and
an endless supply of mints. We aren't supposed to exhaust the students with our bad breath and growling stomachs, the side effects
of our actual bodies.

Some med students get nervous during our encounters. It's like
an awkward date, except half of them are wearing platinum wedding bands. I want to tell them I'm more than just an unmarried
woman faking seizures for pocket money. *I do things!* I want to tell
them. *I'm probably going to write about this in a book someday!* We
make small talk about the rural Iowa farm town I'm supposed to
be from. We each understand the other is inventing this small talk,
and we agree to respond to each other's inventions as genuine ex-
posures of personality. We're holding the fiction between us like a
jump rope.

One time a student forgets we are pretending and starts asking
detailed questions about my fake hometown—which, as it happens,
is his *real* hometown—and his questions lie beyond the purview of
my script, beyond what I can answer, because in truth I don't know
much about the person I'm supposed to be or the place I'm supposed
to be from. He's forgotten our contract. I bullshit harder, more
heartily. "That park in Muscatine!" I say, slapping my knee like a
grandpa. "I used to sled there as a kid."

Other students are all business. They rattle through the clinical
checklist for depression like a list of things they need to get at the
grocery store: *sleep disturbances, changes in appetite, decreased concentration.* Some of them get irritated when I obey my script and refuse to make eye contact. I'm supposed to stay swaddled and numb.
These irritated students take my averted eyes as a challenge. They
never stop seeking my gaze. Wrestling me into eye contact is the
way they maintain power—forcing me to acknowledge their requi-
site display of care.

I grow accustomed to comments that feel aggressive in their for-
mulaic insistence: *that must really be hard* [to have a dying baby], *that*

must really be hard [to be afraid you'll have another seizure in the middle of the grocery store], *that must really be hard* [to carry in your uterus the bacterial evidence of cheating on your husband]. Why not say, *I couldn't even imagine?*

Other students seem to understand that empathy is always perched precariously between gift and invasion. They won't even press the stethoscope to my skin without asking if it's okay. They need permission. They don't want to presume. Their stuttering unwittingly honors my privacy: *Can I . . . could I . . . would you mind if I—listened to your heart?* No, I tell them. I don't mind. Not minding is my job. Their humility is a kind of compassion in its own right. Humility means they ask questions, and questions mean they get answers, and answers mean they get points on the checklist: a point for finding out my mother takes Wellbutrin, a point for getting me to admit I've spent the last two years cutting myself, a point for finding out my father died in a grain elevator when I was two—for realizing that a root system of loss stretches radial and rhyzomatic under the entire territory of my life.

In this sense, empathy isn't just measured by checklist item 31— *voiced empathy for my situation/problem*—but by every item that gauges how thoroughly my experience has been imagined. Empathy isn't just remembering to say *that must really be hard*—it's figuring out how to bring difficulty into the light so it can be seen at all. Empathy isn't just listening, it's asking the questions whose answers need to be listened to. Empathy requires inquiry as much as imagination. Empathy requires knowing you know nothing. Empathy means acknowledging a horizon of context that extends perpetually beyond what you can see: an old woman's gonorrhea is connected to her guilt is connected to her marriage is connected to her children is connected to the days when she was a child. All this is connected to her domestically stifled mother, in turn, and to her parents' unbroken marriage; maybe everything traces its roots to her very first period, how it shamed and thrilled her.

Empathy means realizing no trauma has discrete edges. Trauma bleeds. Out of wounds and across boundaries. Sadness becomes a seizure. Empathy demands another kind of porousness in response. My Stephanie script is twelve pages long. I think mainly about what it doesn't say.

Empathy comes from the Greek *empatheia*—*em* (into) and *pathos* (feeling)—a penetration, a kind of travel. It suggests you enter another person's pain as you'd enter another country, through immigration and customs, border crossing by way of query: *What grows where you are? What are the laws? What animals graze there?*

I've thought about Stephanie Phillips's seizures in terms of possession and privacy. Converting her sadness away from direct articulation is a way to keep it hers. Her refusal to make eye contact, her unwillingness to explicate her inner life, the way she becomes unconscious during her own expressions of grief and doesn't remember them afterward—all of these might be a way to keep her loss protected and pristine, unviolated by the sympathy of others.

"What do you call out during seizures?" one student asks.

"I don't know," I say, and want to add, *but I mean all of it.*

I know that saying this would be against the rules. I'm playing a girl who keeps her sadness so subterranean she can't even see it herself. I can't give it away so easily.

LESLIE JAMISON
Ob-Gyn
SP Training Materials

CASE SUMMARY: You are a twenty-five-year-old female seeking termination of your pregnancy. You have never been pregnant before. You are five-and-a-half weeks but have not experienced any bloating or cramping. You have experienced some fluctuations in mood but have been unable to determine whether these are due to being pregnant or knowing you are pregnant. You are not visibly upset about your pregnancy. Invisibly, you are not sure.

MEDICATION HISTORY: You are not taking any medications. This is why you got pregnant.

MEDICAL HISTORY: You've had several surgeries in the past, but you don't mention them to your doctor because they don't seem relevant. You are about to have another surgery to correct your tachycardia, the excessive and irregular beating of your heart. Your mother has made you promise to mention this upcoming surgery in your termination consultation, even though you don't feel like discussing it. She wants the doctor to know about your heart condition in case it affects the way he ends your pregnancy, or the way he keeps you sedated while he does it.

I could tell you I got an abortion one February or heart surgery that March—like they were separate cases, unrelated scripts—but neither one of these accounts would be complete without the other. A single month knitted them together; each one a morning I woke up on an empty stomach and slid into a paper gown. One depended on a tiny vacuum, the other on a catheter that would ablate the tissue of my heart. *Ablate?* I asked the doctors. They explained that meant burning.

One procedure made me bleed and the other was nearly bloodless; one was my choice and the other wasn't; both made me feel—at once—the incredible frailty and capacity of my own body; both came in a bleak winter; both left me prostrate under the hands of men, and dependent on the care of a man I was just beginning to love.

Dave and I first kissed in a Maryland basement at three in the morning on our way to Newport News to canvass for Obama in 2008. We were with an organizing union called Unite Here. *Unite Here!* Years later, that poster hung above our bed. That first fall we walked along Connecticut beaches strewn with broken clamshells. We held hands against salt winds. We went to a hotel for the weekend and put so much bubble bath in our tub that the bubbles ran all over the floor. We took pictures of that. We took pictures of everything. We walked across Williamsburg in the rain to see a concert. We were writers in love. My boss used to imagine us curling up at night and taking inventories of each other's hearts. "How did it

make you feel to see that injured pigeon in the street today?" etc.
And it's true: we once talked about seeing two crippled bunnies trying to mate on a patchy lawn—how sad it was, and moving.

We'd been in love about two months when I got pregnant. I saw
the cross on the stick and called Dave and we wandered college quads
in the bitter cold and talked about what we were going to do. I thought
of the little fetus bundled inside my jacket with me and wondered—
honestly *wondered*—if I felt attached to it yet. I wasn't sure. I remember not knowing what to say. I remember wanting a drink. I remember
wanting Dave to be inside the choice with me but also feeling posses-
sive of what was happening. I needed him to understand he would
never live this choice like I was going to live it. This was the double
blade of how I felt about anything that hurt: I wanted someone else to
feel it with me, and also I wanted it entirely for myself.

We scheduled the abortion for a Friday, and I found myself facing a week of ordinary days until it happened. I realized I was supposed to keep doing ordinary things. One afternoon, I holed up in
the library and read a pregnancy memoir. The author described a
pulsing fist of fear and loneliness inside her—a fist she'd carried her
whole life, had numbed with drinking and sex—and explained how
her pregnancy had replaced this fist with the tiny bud of her fetus,
a moving life.

I sent Dave a text. I wanted to tell him about the fist of fear,
the baby heart, how sad it felt to read about a woman changed by
her pregnancy when I knew I wouldn't be changed by mine—or at
least, not like she'd been. I didn't hear anything back for hours. This
bothered me. I felt guilt that I didn't feel more about the abortion;
I felt pissed off at Dave for being elsewhere, for choosing not to do
the tiniest thing when I was going to do the rest of it.

I felt the weight of expectation on every moment—the sense
that the end of this pregnancy was something I *should* feel sad
about, the lurking fear that I never felt sad about what I was supposed to feel sad about, the knowledge that I'd gone through several funerals dry eyed, the hunch that I had a parched interior life

activated only by the need for constant affirmation, nothing more. I wanted Dave to guess what I needed at precisely the same time I needed it. I wanted him to imagine how much small signals of his presence might mean.

That night we roasted vegetables and ate them at my kitchen table. Weeks before, I'd covered that table with citrus fruits and fed our friends pills made from berries that made everything sweet: grapefruit tasted like candy, beer like chocolate, Shiraz like Manischewitz— everything, actually, tasted a little like Manischewitz. Which is to say: that kitchen held the ghosts of countless days that felt easier than the one we were living now. We drank wine, and I think—I know—I drank a lot. It sickened me to think I was doing something harmful to the fetus because that meant thinking of the fetus as harmable, which made it feel more alive, which made me feel more selfish, woozy with cheap Cabernet and spoiling for a fight.

Feeling Dave's distance that day had made me realize how much I needed to feel he was as close to this pregnancy as I was—an impossible asymptote. But I thought he could at least bridge the gap between our days and bodies with a text. I told him so. Actually I probably sulked, waited for him to ask, and then told him so. *Guessing your feelings is like charming a cobra with a stethoscope,* another boyfriend told me once. Meaning what? Meaning a few things, I think—that pain turned me venomous, that diagnosing me required a specialized kind of enchantment, that I flaunted feelings and withheld their origins at once.

Sitting with Dave, in my attic living room, my cobra hood was spread. "I felt lonely today," I told him. "I wanted to hear from you."

I'd be lying if I wrote that I remember exactly what he said. I don't. Which is the sad half life of arguments—we usually remember our side better. I think he told me he'd been thinking of me all day, and couldn't I trust that? Why did I need proof?

Voiced concern for my situation/problem. Why did I need proof? I just did.

He said to me, "I think you're making this up."

This meaning what? My anger? My anger at him? Memory fumbles.

I didn't know what I felt, I told him. Couldn't he just trust that I felt something, and that I'd wanted something from him? I needed his empathy not just to comprehend the emotions I was describing, but to help me discover which emotions were actually there.

We were under a skylight under a moon. It was February beyond the glass. It was almost Valentine's Day. I was curled into a cheap futon with crumbs in its creases, a piece of furniture that made me feel like I was still in college. This abortion was something adult. I didn't feel like an adult inside of it.

I heard *making this up* as an accusation that I was inventing emotions I didn't have, but I think he was suggesting I'd mistranslated emotions that were actually there, had been there for a while—that I was attaching long-standing feelings of need and insecurity to the particular event of this abortion; exaggerating what I felt in order to manipulate him into feeling bad. This accusation hurt not because it was entirely wrong but because it was partially right, and because it was leveled with such coldness. He was speaking something truthful about me in order to defend himself, not to make me feel better.

But there was truth behind it. He understood my pain as something actual and constructed at once. He got that it was necessarily both—that my feelings were also made of the way I spoke them. When he told me I was making things up, he didn't mean I wasn't feeling anything. He meant that feeling something was never simply a state of submission but always, also, a process of construction. I see all this, looking back.

I also see that he could have been gentler with me. We could have been gentler with each other.

We went to Planned Parenthood on a freezing morning. We rummaged through a bin of free kids' books while I waited for my name to get called. Who knows why these books were there? Meant for kids waiting during their mothers' appointments, maybe. But it felt like perversity that Friday morning, during the weekly time slot for abortions. We found a book called *Alexander*, about a boy who confesses all his misdeeds to his father by blaming them on an imaginary red-and-green striped horse. *Alexander was a pretty bad horse today.* Whatever we can't hold, we hang on a hook that will hold it. The book belonged to a guy named Michael from Branford. I wondered why Michael had come to Planned Parenthood, and why he'd left that book behind.

There are things I'd like to tell the version of myself who sat in the Planned Parenthood counseling room. I would tell her she is going through something large and she shouldn't be afraid to confess its size, shouldn't be afraid she's "making too big a deal of it." She shouldn't be afraid of not feeling enough because the feelings will keep coming—different ones—for years. I would tell her that commonality doesn't inoculate against hurt. The fact of all those women in the waiting room, doing the same thing I was doing, didn't make it any easier.

I would tell myself: maybe your prior surgeries don't matter here, but maybe they do. Your broken jaw and your broken nose don't have anything to do with your pregnancy except they were both times you got broken into. Getting each one fixed meant getting broken into again. Getting your heart fixed will be another burglary, nothing taken except everything that gets burned away. Maybe every time you get into a paper gown you summon the ghosts of all the other times you got into a paper gown; maybe every time you slip down into that anesthetized dark it's the same dark you slipped into before. Maybe it's been waiting for you the whole time.

STEPHANIE PHILLIPS
Psychiatry
SP Training Materials (Cont.)

OPENING LINE: "I'm having these seizures and no one knows why."

PHYSICAL PRESENTATION AND TONE: You are wearing jeans and a sweatshirt, preferably stained or rumpled. You aren't someone who puts much effort into your personal appearance. At some point during the encounter, you might mention that you don't bother dressing nicely anymore because you rarely leave the house. It is essential that you avoid eye contact and keep your voice free of emotion during the encounter.

One of the hardest parts of playing Stephanie Phillips is nailing her affect—*la belle indifférence,* a manner defined as the "air of unconcern displayed by some patients toward their physical symptoms." It is a common sign of conversion disorder, a front of indifference hiding "physical symptoms [that] may relieve anxiety and result in secondary gains in the form of sympathy and attention given by others." *La belle indifférence*—outsourcing emotional content to physical expression—is a way of inviting empathy without asking for it. In this way, encounters with Stephanie present a sort of empathy limit case: the clinician must excavate a sadness the patient hasn't identified, must imagine a pain Stephanie can't fully experience herself.

For other cases, we are supposed to wear our anguish more openly—like a terrible, seething garment. My first time playing Appendicitis Angela, I'm told I manage "just the right amount of pain." I'm moaning in a fetal position and apparently doing it right. The doctors know how to respond. "I am sorry to hear that you are experiencing an excruciating pain in your abdomen," one says. "It must be uncomfortable."

Part of me has always craved a pain so visible—so irrefutable and physically inescapable—that everyone would have to notice. But my sadness about the abortion was never a convulsion. There was never a scene. No frothing at the mouth. I was almost relieved, three days after the procedure, when I started to hurt. It was worst at night, the cramping. But at least I knew what I felt. I wouldn't have to figure out how to explain. Like Stephanie, who didn't talk about her grief because her seizures were already pronouncing it— slantwise, in a private language, but still—granting it substance and choreography.

STEPHANIE PHILLIPS

Psychiatry

SP Training Materials (Cont.)

ENCOUNTER DYNAMICS: You don't reveal personal details until prompted. You wouldn't call yourself happy. You wouldn't call yourself unhappy. You get sad some nights about your brother. You don't say so. You don't say you have a turtle who might outlive you, and a pair of green sneakers from your gig at the minigolf course. You don't say you have a lot of memories of stacking putters. You say you have another brother, if asked, but you don't say he's not Will, because that's obvious—even if the truth of it still strikes you sometimes, hard. You're not sure these things matter. They're just facts. They're facts like the fact of dried spittle on your cheeks when you wake up on the couch and can't remember telling your mother to fuck herself. *Fuck you* is also what your arm says when it jerks so hard it might break into pieces. *Fuck you fuck you fuck you* until your jaw locks and nothing comes.

You live in a world underneath the words you are saying in this clean white room, *it's okay I'm okay I feel sad I guess.* You are blind in this other world. It's dark. Your seizures are how you move through it— thrashing and fumbling—feeling for what its walls are made of.

Your body wasn't anything special until it rebelled. Maybe you thought your thighs were fat or else you didn't, yet; maybe you had best friends who whispered secrets to you during sleepovers; maybe you had lots of boyfriends or else you were still waiting for the first one; maybe you liked unicorns when you were young or maybe you preferred regular horses. I imagine you in every possible direction, and then I cover my tracks and imagine you all over again. Sometimes I can't stand how much of you I don't know.

I hadn't planned to get heart surgery right after my abortion. I hadn't planned to get heart surgery at all. It came as a surprise that there was anything wrong. My pulse had been showing up high at the doctor's office. I was given a Holter monitor—a small plastic box to wear around my neck for twenty-four hours, attached by

sensors to my chest—that showed the doctors my heart wasn't beating right. The doctors diagnosed me with SVT—supraventricular
tachycardia—and said they thought there was an extra electrical
node sending out extra signals—*beat, beat, beat*—when it wasn't
supposed to.

They explained how to fix it: they'd make two slits in my skin,
above my hips, and thread catheter wires all the way up to my heart.
They would ablate bits of tissue until they managed to get rid of my
tiny rogue beat box.

My primary cardiologist was a small woman who moved quickly
through the offices and hallways of her world. Let's call her Dr. M.
She spoke in a curt voice, always. The problem was never that her
curtness meant anything—never that I took it personally—but
rather that it meant nothing, that it wasn't personal at all.

My mother insisted I call Dr. M. to tell her I was having an
abortion. What if there was something I needed to tell the doctors
before they performed it? That was the reasoning. I put off the call
until I couldn't put it off any longer. The thought of telling a near-
stranger that I was having an abortion—over the phone, without
being asked—seemed mortifying. It was like I'd be peeling off the
bandage on a wound she hadn't asked to see.

When I finally got her on the phone, she sounded harried and
impatient. I told her quickly. Her voice was cold: "And what do you
want to know from me?"

I went blank. I hadn't known I'd wanted her to say *I'm sorry
to hear that* until she didn't say it. But I had. I'd wanted her to say
something. I started crying. I felt like a child. I felt like an idiot.
Why was I crying now, when I hadn't cried before—not when I
found out, not when I told Dave, not when I made the consultation
appointment or went to it?

"Well?" she asked.

I finally remembered my question: did the abortion doctor need
to know anything about my tachycardia?

"No," she said. There was a pause, and then: "Is that it?" Her
voice was so incredibly blunt. I could only hear one thing in it:

Why are you making a fuss? That was it. I felt simultaneously like I didn't feel enough and like I was making a big deal out of nothing—that maybe I was making a big deal out of nothing *because* I didn't feel enough, that my tears with Dr. M. were runoff from the other parts of the abortion I wasn't crying about. I had an insecurity that didn't know how to express itself; that could attach itself to tears or to their absence. *Alexander was a pretty bad horse today.* When of course the horse wasn't the problem. Dr. M. became a villain because my story didn't have one. It was the kind of pain that comes without a perpetrator. Everything was happening because of my body or because of a choice I'd made. I needed something from the world I didn't know how to ask for. I needed people—Dave, a doctor, anyone—to deliver my feelings back to me in a form that was legible. Which is a superlative kind of empathy to seek, or to supply: an empathy that rearticulates more clearly what it's shown.

A month later, Dr. M. bent over the operating table and apologized. "I'm sorry for my tone on the phone," she said. "When you called about your abortion. I didn't understand what you were asking." It was an apology whose logic I didn't entirely follow. *(Didn't understand what you were asking?)* It was an apology that had been prompted. At some point my mother had called Dr. M. to discuss my upcoming procedure—and had mentioned I'd been upset by our conversation.

Now I was lying on my back in a hospital gown. I was woozy from the early stages of my anesthesia. I felt like crying all over again, at the memory of how powerless I'd been on the phone—powerless because I needed so much from her, a stranger—and at a sense of how powerless I was now, lying flat on my back and waiting for a team of doctors to burn away the tissue of my heart. I wanted to tell her I didn't accept her apology. I wanted to tell her she didn't have the right to apologize—not here, not while I was lying naked under a paper gown, not when I was about to get cut open again. I wanted to deny her the right to feel better because she'd said she was sorry.

Mainly, I wanted the anesthesia to carry me away from everything I felt and everything my body was about to feel. In a moment,
it did.

I always fight the impulse to ask the med students for pills during our
encounters. It seems natural. Wouldn't Baby Doug's mom want an
Ativan? Wouldn't Appendicitis Angela want some Vicodin, or whatever they give you for a ten on the pain scale? Wouldn't Stephanie
Phillips be a little more excited about a new diet of Valium? I keep
thinking I'll communicate my pain most effectively by expressing
my desire for the things that might dissolve it. If I were Stephanie
Phillips, I'd be excited about my Ativan. But I'm not. And being an
SP isn't about projection; it's about inhabitance. I can't go off script.
These encounters aren't about dissolving pain. They're about seeing
it more clearly. The healing part is always a hypothetical horizon we
never reach.

During my winter of ministrations, I found myself constantly in
the hands of doctors. It began with that first nameless man who
gave me an abortion the same morning he gave twenty other women
their abortions. Gave. It's a funny word we use, as if it were a present. Once the procedure was done, I was wheeled into a dim room
where a man with a long white beard gave me a cup of orange juice.
He was like a kid's drawing of God. I remember resenting how he
wouldn't give me any pain pills until I'd eaten a handful of crackers,
but he was kind. His resistance was a kind of care. I felt that. He
was looking out for me.

Dr. G. was the doctor who performed my heart operation. He
controlled the catheters from a remote computer. It looked like a
spaceship flight cabin. He had a nimble voice and lanky arms and
bushy white hair. I liked him. He was a straight talker. He came
into the hospital room the day after my operation and explained
why the procedure hadn't worked: they'd burned and burned, but
they hadn't burned the right patch. They'd even cut through my ar-

terial wall to keep looking. But then they'd stopped. Ablating more tissue risked dismantling my circuitry entirely.

Dr. G. said I could get the procedure again. I could authorize them to ablate more aggressively. The risk was that I'd come out of surgery with a pacemaker. He was very calm when he said this. He pointed at my chest: "On someone thin," he said, "you'd be able to see the outlines of the box quite clearly."

I pictured waking up from general anesthesia to find a metal box above my ribs. I remember being struck by how the doctor had anticipated a question about the pacemaker I hadn't yet discovered in myself: How easily would I be able to forget it was there? I remember feeling grateful for the calmness in his voice and not offended by it. It didn't register as callousness. Why?

Maybe it was just because he was a man. I didn't need him to be my mother—even for a day—I only needed him to know what he was doing. But I think it was something more. Instead of identifying with my panic—inhabiting my horror at the prospect of a pacemaker— he was helping me understand that even this, the barnacle of a false heart, would be okay. His calmness didn't make me feel abandoned, it made me feel secure. It offered assurance rather than empathy, or maybe assurance was evidence of empathy, insofar as he understood that assurance, not identification, was what I needed most.

Empathy is a kind of care but it's not the only kind of care, and it's not always enough. I want to think that's what Dr. G. was thinking. I needed to look at him and see the opposite of my fear, not its echo.

Every time I met with Dr. M., she began our encounters with a few perfunctory questions about my life—*What are you working on these days?*—and when she left the room to let me dress, I could hear her voice speaking into a tape recorder in the hallway: *Patient is a graduate student in English at Yale. Patient is writing a dissertation on addiction. Patient spent two years living in Iowa. Patient is working on a collection of essays.* And then, without fail, at the next appointment, fresh from listening to her old tape, she bullet-pointed a few questions: *How were those two years in Iowa? How's that collection of essays?*

It was a strange intimacy, almost embarrassing, to feel the mechanics of her method so palpable between us: *engage the patient, record the details, repeat.* I was sketched into CliffsNotes. I hated seeing the puppet strings; they felt unseemly—and without kindness in her voice, the mechanics meant nothing. They pretended we knew each other rather than acknowledging that we didn't. It's a tension intrinsic to the surgeon-patient relationship: it's more invasive than anything but not intimate at all.

Now I can imagine another kind of tape—a more naked, stuttering tape; a tape that keeps correcting itself, that messes up its dance steps:

Patient is here ~~for an abortion~~ for ~~a surgery to burn the bad parts of her heart~~ for a medication to fix her heart because the surgery failed. Patient is staying in the hospital for ~~one night~~ ~~three nights~~ five nights until we get this medication right. Patient ~~wonders if people can bring her booze in the hospital~~ likes to eat graham crackers from the nurses' station. Patient cannot be released until she runs on a treadmill and her heart prints a clean rhythm. Patient recently got an abortion but we don't understand why she wanted us to know that. Patient didn't ~~think she~~ hurt at first but then she did. Patient ~~failed to use protection and~~ failed to provide an adequate account of why she didn't use protection. ~~Patient had a lot of feelings. Partner of patient had the feeling she was making up a lot of feelings.~~ Partner of patient is supportive. Partner of patient is spotted in patient's hospital bed, repeatedly. Partner of patient is caught kissing patient. Partner of patient is charming.

Patient is ~~angry~~ ~~disappointed~~ angry her procedure failed. Patient does not want to be on medication. Patient wants to know if she can drink alcohol on this medication. She wants to know how much. She wants to know ~~if two bottles of wine a night is too much~~ if she can get away with a couple of glasses. Patient does not want to get another procedure if it means risking a pacemaker. Patient wants everyone to understand that this surgery ~~is~~ isn't a big deal; wants everyone to understand she is stupid for crying when everyone else on the ward is sicker than she is; wants everyone to understand her abortion is ~~also about~~ definitely not about the children her ex-boyfriends have had since she broke up with them. Patient wants everyone to understand ~~it wasn't a choice~~ it would have been easier if it hadn't been a choice. Patient understands it was her choice to drink while she was pregnant. She understands it was her choice to go to a bar with a little plastic box hanging from her neck, and get so drunk she messed up her heart graph. Patient is patients, plural, meaning she is multiple—mostly grateful but sometimes surly, sometimes full of self-pity. Patient ~~already understands~~ is trying hard to understand she needs to listen up if she wants to hear how everyone is caring for her.

Three men waited for me in the hospital during my surgery: my brother and my father and Dave. They sat in the lounge making awkward conversation, and then in the cafeteria making awkward conversation, and then—I'm not sure where they sat, actually, or in what order, because I wasn't there. But I do know that while they were sitting in the cafeteria a doctor came to find them and told them that the surgeons were going to tear through part of my arterial wall—these were the words they used, Dave said, *tear through*—and try burning some patches of tissue on the other side. At this point, Dave told me later, he went to the hospital chapel and prayed I wouldn't die. He prayed in the nook made by the propped-open door because he didn't want to be seen.

It wasn't likely I would die. Dave didn't know that then. Prayer isn't about likelihood anyway, it's about desire—loving someone enough to get on your knees and ask for her to be saved. When he cried in that chapel, it wasn't empathy—it was something else. His kneeling wasn't a way to feel my pain but to request that it end.

I learned to rate Dave on how well he empathized with me. I was constantly poised above an invisible checklist item 31. I wanted him to hurt whenever I hurt, to feel as much as I felt. But it's exhausting to keep tabs on how much someone is feeling for you. It can make you forget that they feel too.

I used to believe that hurting would make you more alive to the hurting of others. I used to believe in feeling bad because somebody else did. Now I'm not so sure of either. I know that being in the hospital made me selfish. Getting surgeries made me think mainly about whether I'd have to get another one. When bad things happened to other people, I imagined them happening to me. I didn't know if this was empathy or theft.

For example: one September, my brother woke up in a hotel room in Sweden and couldn't move half his face. He was diagnosed with something called Bell's palsy. No one really understands why it happens or how to make it better. The doctors gave him a steroid called prednisone that made him sick. He threw up most days around twilight. He sent us a photo. It looked lonely and grainy. His face slumped. His pupil glistened in the flash, bright with the gel he had to put on his eye to keep it from drying out. He couldn't blink.

I found myself obsessed with his condition. I tried to imagine what it was like to move through the world with an unfamiliar face. I thought about what it would be like to wake up in the morning, in the groggy space where you've managed to forget things, to forget your whole life, and then snapping to, realizing: *yes, this is how things are.* Checking the mirror: still there. I tried to imagine how you'd feel a little crushed, each time, coming out of dreams to another day of being awake with a face not quite your own.

I spent large portions of each day—pointless, fruitless spans of time—imagining how I would feel if my face was paralyzed too. I stole my brother's trauma and projected it onto myself like a magic-lantern pattern of light. I obsessed, and told myself this obsession was empathy. But it wasn't, quite. It was more like *in*pathy. I wasn't expatriating myself into another life so much as importing its problems into my own.

Dave doesn't believe in feeling bad just because someone else does. This isn't his notion of support. He believes in listening, and asking questions, and steering clear of assumptions. He thinks imagining someone else's pain with too much surety can be as damaging as failing to imagine it. He believes in humility. He believes in stay-

ing strong enough to stick around. He stayed with me in the hospital, five nights in those crisp white beds, and he lay down with
my monitor wires, colored strands carrying the electrical signature
of my heart to a small box I held in my hands. I remember lying
tangled with him, how much it meant—that he was willing to lie
down in the mess of wires, to stay there with me.

In order to help the med students empathize better with us, we have
to empathize with them. I try to think about what makes them fall
short of what they're asked—what nervousness or squeamishness
or callousness—and how to speak to their sore spots without bruising them: the one so stiff he shook my hand like we'd just made a
business deal; the chipper one so eager to befriend me she didn't
wash her hands at all.

One day we have a sheet cake delivered for my supervisor's
birthday—dry white layers with ripples of strawberry jelly—and
we sit around our conference table eating her cake with plastic forks
while she doesn't eat anything at all. She tells us what kind of syntax we should use when we tell the students about bettering their
empathy. We're supposed to use the "When you . . . I felt" frame.
*When you forgot to wash your hands, I felt protective of my body. When
you told me eleven wasn't on the pain scale, I felt dismissed.* For the
good parts also: *When you asked me questions about Will, I felt like
you really cared about my loss.*

A 1983 study titled "The Structure of Empathy" found a correla-
tion between empathy and four major personality clusters: sensitivity, nonconformity, even temperedness, and social self-confidence. I
like the word *structure*. It suggests empathy is an edifice we build like
a home or office—with architecture and design, scaffolding and electricity. The Chinese character for *listen* is built like this, a structure
of many parts: the characters for ears and eyes, a horizontal line that
signifies undivided attention, the swoop and teardrops of heart.

Rating high for the study's "sensitivity" cluster feels intuitive. It
means agreeing with statements like "I have at one time or another
tried my hand at writing poetry" or "I have seen some things so sad

they almost made me feel like crying" and *dis*agreeing with statements like: "I really don't care whether people like me or dislike me." This last one seems to suggest that empathy might be, at root, a barter, a bid for others' affection: *I care about your pain* is another way to say *I care if you like me.* We care in order to be cared for. We care because we are porous. The feelings of others matter, they are *like* matter: they carry weight, exert gravitational pull.

It's the last cluster, social self-confidence, that I don't understand as well. I've always treasured empathy as the particular privilege of the invisible, the observers who are shy precisely *because* they sense so much—because it is overwhelming to say even a single word when you're sensitive to every last flicker of nuance in the room. "The relationship between social self-confidence and empathy is the most difficult to understand," the study admits. But its explanation makes sense: social confidence is a prerequisite but not a guarantee; it can "give a person the courage to enter the interpersonal world and practice empathetic skills." We should empathize from courage, is the point—and it makes me think about how much of my empathy comes from fear. I'm afraid other people's problems will happen to me, or else I'm afraid other people will stop loving me if I don't adopt their problems as my own.

Jean Decety, a psychologist at the University of Chicago, uses fMRI scans to measure what happens when someone's brain responds to another person's pain. He shows test subjects images of painful situations (hand caught in scissors, foot under door) and compares these scans to what a brain looks like when its body is actually in pain. Decety has found that imagining the pain of others activates the same three areas (prefrontal cortex, anterior insula, anterior cingulate) as experiencing pain itself. I feel heartened by that correspondence. But I also wonder what it's good for.

During the months of my brother's Bell's palsy, whenever I woke up in the morning and checked my face for a fallen cheek, a drooping eye, a collapsed smile, I wasn't ministering to anyone. I wasn't feeling toward my brother so much as I was feeling toward a version of myself—a self that didn't exist but theoretically shared his misfortune.

I wonder if my empathy has always been this, in every case: just a bout of hypothetical self-pity projected onto someone else. Is this ultimately just solipsism? Adam Smith confesses in his *Theory of Moral Sentiments:* "When we see a stroke aimed and just ready to fall upon the leg or arm of another person, we naturally shrink and draw back our own leg or our own arm."

We care about ourselves. Of course we do. Maybe some good comes from it. If I imagine myself fiercely into my brother's pain, I get some sense, perhaps, of what he might want or need, because I think, *I would want this. I would need this.* But it also seems like a fragile pretext, turning his misfortunes into an opportunity to indulge pet fears of my own devising.

I wonder which parts of my brain are lighting up when the med students ask me: "How does that make you feel?" Or which parts of their brains are glowing when I say, "The pain in my abdomen is a ten." My condition isn't real. I know this. They know this. I'm simply going through the motions. They're simply going through the motions. But motions can be more than rote. They don't just express feeling; they can give birth to it.

Empathy isn't just something that happens to us—a meteor shower of synapses firing across the brain—it's also a choice we make: to pay attention, to extend ourselves. It's made of exertion, that dowdier cousin of impulse. Sometimes we care for another because we know we should, or because it's asked for, but this doesn't make our caring hollow. The act of choosing simply means we've committed ourselves to a set of behaviors greater than the sum of our individual inclinations: *I will listen to his sadness, even when I'm deep in my own.* To say *going through the motions*—this isn't reduction so much as acknowledgment of effort—the labor, the *motions,* the dance—of getting inside another person's state of heart or mind.

This confession of effort chafes against the notion that empathy should always rise unbidden, that *genuine* means the same thing as *unwilled,* that intentionality is the enemy of love. But I believe in intention and I believe in work. I believe in waking up in the middle

of the night and packing our bags and leaving our worst selves for
our better ones.

LESLIE JAMISON
Ob-Gyn
SP Training Materials (Cont.)

OPENING LINE: You don't need one. Everyone comes here for the
same reason.

PHYSICAL PRESENTATION AND TONE: Wear loose pants. You have
been told to wear loose pants. Keep your voice steady and articulate.
You are about to spread your legs for a doctor who won't ever know
your name. You know the drill, sort of. Act like you do.

ENCOUNTER DYNAMICS: Answer every question like you're clarifying
a coffee order. Be courteous and nod vigorously. Make sure your heart
stays on the other side of the white wall behind you. If the nurse asks
you whether you are sure about getting the procedure, say *yes* without
missing a beat. Say *yes* without a trace of doubt. Don't mention the
way you felt when you first saw the pink cross on the stick—that sudden
expansive joy at the possibility of a child, at your own capacity to have
one. Don't mention this single moment of joy because it might make it
seem as if you aren't completely sure about what you're about to do.
Don't mention this single moment of joy because it might hurt. It will
feel—more than anything else does—like the measure of what you're
giving up. It maps the edges of your voluntary loss.

　　Instead, tell the nurse you weren't using birth control but wasn't that
silly and now you are going to start.

　　If she asks what forms of birth control you have used in the past,
say condoms. Suddenly every guy you've ever slept with is in the room
with you. Ignore them. Ignore the memory of that first time—all that
fumbling, and then pain—while Rod Stewart crooned "Broken Arrow"
from a boom box on the dresser. *Who else is gonna bring you a broken
arrow? Who else is gonna bring you a bottle of rain?*

　　Say you used condoms but don't think about all the times you didn't—in an Iowan graveyard, in a little car by a dark river—and definitely don't say why, how the risk made you feel close to those boys, how you courted the incredible gravity of what your bodies could do together.

If the nurse asks about your current partner, you should say, *we are very committed,* like you are defending yourself against some legal charge. If the nurse is listening closely, she should hear fear nestled like an egg inside your certainty.

If the nurse asks whether you drink, say *yes* to that too. Of course you do. Like it's no big deal. Your lifestyle habits include drinking to excess. You do this even when you know there is a fetus inside you. You do it to forget there is a fetus inside you; or to feel like maybe this is just a movie about a fetus being inside you.

The nurse will eventually ask, *how do you feel about getting the procedure?* Tell her you feel sad but you know it's the right choice, because this seems like the right thing to say, even though it's a lie. You feel mainly numb. You feel numb until your legs are in the stirrups. Then you hurt. Whatever anesthesia comes through the needle in your arm only sedates you. Days later you feel your body cramping in the night— a deep, hot, twisting pain—and you can only lie still and hope it passes, beg for sleep, drink for sleep, resent Dave for sleeping next to you. You can only watch your body bleed like an inscrutable, stubborn object— something harmed and cumbersome and not entirely yours. You leave your body and don't come back for a month. You come back angry.

You wake up from another round of anesthesia and they tell you all their burning didn't burn away the part of your heart that was broken. You come back and find you aren't alone. You weren't alone when you were cramping through the night and you're not alone now. Dave spends every night in the hospital. You want to tell him how disgusting your body feels: your unwashed skin and greasy hair. You want him to listen, for hours if necessary, and feel everything exactly as you feel it—your pair of hearts in such synchronized rhythm any monitor would show it; your pair of hearts playing two crippled bunnies doing whatever they can. There is no end to this fantasy of closeness. *Who else is gonna bring you a broken arrow?* You want him to break with you. You want him to hurt in a womb he doesn't have; you want him to admit he can't hurt that way. You want him to know how it feels in every one of your nerve endings: lying prone on the detergent sheets, lifting your shirt for one more cardiac resident, one more stranger, letting him attach his clips to the line of hooks under your breast, letting him print out your heart, once more, to see if its rhythm has calmed.

It all returns to this: you want him close to your damage. You want humility and presumption and whatever lies between, you want that too. You're tired of begging for it. You're tired of grading him on how well he gives it. You want to learn how to stop feeling sorry for yourself. You want to write an essay about the lesson. You throw away the checklist and let him climb into your hospital bed. You let him part the heart wires. You sleep. He sleeps. You wake, pulse feeling for another pulse, and there he is again.

‡ DEVIL'S BAIT ‡

Introduction

For Paul, it started with a fishing trip. For Lenny, it was an addict whose knuckles were covered in sores. Dawn found pimples clustered around her swimming goggles. Kendra noticed ingrown hairs. Patricia was attacked by sand flies on a Gulf Coast beach. The sickness can start as blisters, or lesions, or itching, or simply a terrible fog settling over the mind, over the world.

For me, Morgellons disease started as a novelty: people said they had a strange disease, and no one—or hardly anyone—believed them. But there were a lot of them, almost twelve thousand of them, and their numbers were growing. Their illness manifested in lots of ways: sores, itching, fatigue, pain, and something called formication, the sensation of crawling insects. But its defining symptom was always the same: strange fibers emerging from underneath the skin.

In short, people were finding unidentifiable matter coming out of their bodies. Not just fibers but fuzz, specks, and crystals. They didn't know what this matter was, or where it came from, or why it was there, but they knew—and this was what mattered, the important word—that it was *real*.

The diagnosis originated with a woman named Mary Leitao. In 2001, she took her toddler son to the doctor because he had sores on his lip that wouldn't go away. He was complaining of bugs under his skin. The first doctor didn't know what to tell her, and neither did the second, or the third. Eventually, they started telling her something she didn't want to hear: that she might be suffering from Munchausen syndrome by proxy, because they couldn't find anything wrong with her son. Leitao came up with her own diagnosis; Morgellons was born.

Leitao pulled the name from a treatise written by a seventeenth-century doctor named Thomas Browne:

> I long ago observed in that Endemial Distemper of little Children in Languedock, called the Morgellons, wherein they critically break out with harsh Hairs on their Backs, which takes off the Unquiet Symptomes of the Disease, and delivers them from Coughs and Convulsions.

Browne's "harsh hairs" were the early ancestors of today's fibers, the threads that form the core of this disease. Magnified photos online show them in red, white, and blue—like the flag—and also black and clear. These fibers are the kind of thing you describe in relation to other kinds of things: jellyfish or wires, animal fur or taffy candy or a fuzz ball off your grandma's sweater. Some are called "goldenheads" because they have a golden-colored bulb. Others look like cobras curling out of the skin, thread-thin but ready to strike. Others simply look sinister, technological, tangled. The magnification in these photos makes it hard to know what you're looking at; if you're even seeing skin.

Patients started bringing these threads and flecks and fuzz to their doctors, storing them in Tupperware or matchboxes, and dermatologists actually developed a phrase for this: "the matchbox sign," a signal that the patient had become so determined to prove his own disease that he could no longer be trusted.

By the mid-2000s, Morgellons had become a controversy in earnest. Self-identified patients started calling themselves "Morgies" and rallying against doctors who diagnosed them with something called delusions of parasitosis (DOP). The CDC launched a full-scale investigation in 2006. Major newspapers published articles: "Is It Disease or Delusion?" (*New York Times*); "CDC Probes Bizarre

Morgellons Condition" (*Boston Globe*); "Curious, Controversial Disease Morgellons Confounding Patients, Doctors Alike" (*Los Angeles Times*).

In the meantime, a Morgellons advocacy organization called the Charles E. Holman Foundation started putting together an annual conference in Austin for patients, researchers, and health care providers—basically, anyone who gave a damn. The foundation was named for a man who devoted the last years of his life to investigating the causes of his wife's disease. His widow still runs the gathering. She's still sick. The conference offers refuge—to her and others—from a world that generally refuses to accept their account of why they suffer. As one presenter wrote to me by e-mail:

> It is bad enough that people are suffering so terribly. But to be the topic of seemingly the biggest joke in the world is way too much for sick people to bear. It is amazing to me that more people with this dreadful illness do not commit suicide . . . The story is even more bizarre than you may realize. Morgellons is a perfect storm of an illness, complete with heroes, villains, and very complex people trying to do what they think is right.

The CDC finally released the results of its study "Clinical, Epidemiologic, Histopathologic and Molecular Features of an Unexplained Dermopathy" in January 2012. The report is neatly carved into movements—*Introduction, Methods, Results, Discussion, Acknowledgments*—but it offers no easy conclusions. Its authors, the so-called Unexplained Dermopathy Task Force, investigated 115 patients, using skin samples, blood tests, and neurocognitive exams. Their report offers little comfort to Morgies looking for confirmation: "We were not able to conclude based on this study whether this unexplained dermopathy represents a new condition . . . or wider recognition of an existing condition such as delusional infestation."

The bottom line? Probably nothing there.

Methods

The Westoak Baptist Church, on Slaughter Lane, is a few miles
south of the Austin I'd imagined, a city full of Airstream trailers selling gourmet donuts, vintage shops crammed with animal
heads and lace, melancholy guitar riffs floating from ironic cowboy bars. Slaughter Lane isn't vintage lace or cutting-edge donuts
or ironic anything; it's Walgreens and Denny's and eventually a
parking lot sliced by the spindly shadow of a twenty-foot cross.

The church itself is a low blue building surrounded by temporary
trailers. A conference banner reads: *Searching for the Uncommon
Thread.* I've arrived at the conference in the aftermath of the CDC
report, as the Morgellons community assembles once more—to re-
group, to respond, to insist.

A cluster of friendly women stand by the entrance greeting new
arrivals. They wear matching shirts printed with the letters DOP
slashed by a diagonal red line. Most of the participants at the
conference, I will come to realize, give the wholesome, welcoming
impression of no-nonsense midwestern housewives. I learn that
70 percent of Morgellons patients are female—and that women are
especially vulnerable to the isolating disfigurement and condescension that come attached to the disease.

The greeters direct me past an elaborate buffet of packaged pas-
tries and into the church sanctuary, which is serving as the main
conference room. Speakers stand at the makeshift pulpit (a lectern)
with their PowerPoint slides projected onto a screen behind them.
The stage is cluttered with musical equipment. Each cloth-covered
pew holds a single box of Kleenex. There's a special eating area in
the back: tables littered with coffee cups, muffin-greased plastic,
and the skeletons of grape bunches. The room has one stained-glass
window—a dark blue circle holding the milky cataract of a dove—
but the colors admit no light. The window is small enough to make
the dove look trapped; it's not flying but stuck.

This gathering is something like an AA meeting or a Quaker
service: between speakers, people occasionally just walk up to the

podium and start sharing. Or else they do it in their chairs, hunched over to get a better look at each other's limbs. They swap cell phone photos. I hear a man tell a woman: "I live in a bare apartment near work; don't have much else." I hear her reply: "But you still work?"

Here's what else I hear: "So you just run the sound waves through your feet . . . you see them coming out as chunks, literally hanging off the skin? . . . you got it from your dad? . . . you gave it to your son? . . . My sons are still young . . . he has fibers in his hair but no lesions on his skin . . . I use a teaspoon of salt and a teaspoon of vitamin C . . . I was drinking Borax for a while but I couldn't keep it up . . . HR told me not to talk about it . . . your arms look better than last year . . . you seem better than last year . . . but you feel better than last year?" I hear someone talking about what her skin is "expressing." I hear someone say, "It's a lonely world." I feel close to the specter of whole years lost.

I discover that the people who can't help whispering during lectures are the ones I want to talk to; that the coffee station is useful because it's a good place to meet people, and because drinking coffee means I'll have to keep going to the bathroom, which is an even better place to meet people. The people I meet don't look disfigured at first glance. But up close, they reveal all kinds of scars and bumps and scabs. They are covered in records—fossils or ruins—of the open, oozing things that once were.

I meet Patricia, wearing a periwinkle pantsuit, who tells me how she got attacked by sand flies one summer and everything changed. I meet Shirley, who thinks her family got sick from camping at a tick-rich place called Rocky Neck. Shirley's daughter has been on antibiotics for so long she has to lie to her doctor about why she needs them.

I meet Dawn, an articulate and graceful nurse from Pittsburgh, whose legs show the white patches I've come to recognize as once-scabbed or lesion-ridden skin. Antibiotics left a pattern of dark patches on her calves that once got her mistaken for an AIDS patient. Since diagnosing herself with Morgellons, Dawn has kept her full-time position as a nurse because she wants to direct her frustration into useful work.

"I was so angry at the misdiagnoses for so many years," she says, "being told that it was anxiety, in my head, female stuff. So I tried to spin that anger into something positive. I got my graduate degree; I published an article in a nursing journal."

I ask her about this phrase: *female stuff.* It's like heart disease, she explains. For a long time women's heart attacks went unnoticed because they were diagnosed as symptoms of anxiety. I realize her disease is part of a complicated history that goes all the way back to nineteenth-century hysteria. Dawn says her coworkers—the nurses, not the doctors—have been remarkably empathetic; and she suggests it's no mere coincidence that most of these nurses are women. Now they come to her whenever they find something strange or unexpected in a wound: fuzz or flakes or threads. She's become an expert in the unexplainable.

I ask Dawn what the hardest part of her disease has been. At first she replies in general terms—"Uncertain future?"—lilting her answer into a question, but soon finds her way to a more specific fear: "Afraid of relationships," she says, "because who's gonna accept me?" She continues, her speaking full of pauses: "I just feel very— what's the word . . . not conspicuous, but very . . . with scars and stuff that I have from this, what guy's gonna like me?"

I tell her I don't see a scarred woman when I look at her; I think she's beautiful. She thanks me for saying so, but I can tell the compliment rang a bit hollow. One comment from a stranger can't reclaim years spent hating the body you live in.

With Dawn I fall into the easy groove of identification—*I've felt that too*—whenever she talks about her body as something that's done her wrong. Her condition seems like a crystallization of what I've always felt about myself—a wrongness in my being that I could never pin or name, so I found things to pin it to: my body, my thighs, my face. This resonance is part of what compels me about Morgellons: it offers a shape for what I've often felt, a container or christening for a certain species of unease. Dis-ease. Though I also feel how every attempt to metaphorize the illness is also an act of violence—an argument against the bodily reality its patients insist upon.

My willingness to turn Morgellons into metaphor—as a corporeal manifestation of some abstract human tendency—is dangerous. It obscures the particular and unbidden nature of the suffering
in front of me.

It would be too easy to let all these faces dissolve into correlative
possibility: Morgies as walking emblems for how hard it is for all of
us to live in our own skin. I feel how conveniently these lives could
be sculpted to fit the metaphoric structure—or strictures—of the
essay itself.

A woman named Rita from Memphis, another nurse, talks to me
about doctors—the ones who didn't believe her; the ones who told
her she was out of luck, or out of her mind; the one who happened
to share her surname but slammed a door in her face anyway. She
felt especially wronged by that gesture—the specter of kinship, a
shared name, cast aside so forcefully.

Rita tells me she lost her job and husband because of this disease. She tells me she hasn't had health insurance in years. She tells
me she can literally see her skin moving. Do I believe her? I nod. I
tell myself I can agree with a declaration of pain without being certain I agree with the declaration of its cause.

Rita tells me she handles a Morgellons hotline. People call if they
suspect they might have the disease but don't know much about it. I
ask her what she tells them. She reassures them, she says. She tells
them there are people out there who will believe them.

The most important advice she gives? *Don't take specimens in.*
That's the number one rule, she says. Otherwise they'll think you're
crazy in a heartbeat.

I once had a specimen of my own. It was a worm in my ankle, a
botfly larva I'd brought back from Bolivia. The human botfly lays
its egg on a mosquito proboscis, where it is deposited—via mosquito bite—under the skin. In the Amazon, it's no big deal. In New
Haven, it's less familiar. I saw mine emerge around midnight: a
small pale maggot. That's when I took a cab to the ER. I remember

saying: "There's a worm in there," and I remember how everyone looked at me, doctors and nurses: kindly and without belief. Their doubt was like humidity in the air. They asked me if I'd recently taken any mind-altering drugs. The disconnect felt even worse than the worm itself—to live in a world where this thing *was*, while other people lived in a world where it wasn't.

For weeks, down in Bolivia, I'd been living with the suspicion that I had something living under my skin. It was almost a relief to finally see it, bobbing out of my ankle like a tiny white snorkel. I finally knew it was true. It's Othello's Desdemona Problem: fearing the worst is worse than *knowing* the worst. So you eventually start wanting the worst possible thing to happen—finding your wife in bed with another man, or watching the worm finally come into the light. Until the worst happens, it always *might* happen. When it actually does happen? Now, at least, you know.

I remember the shrill intensity of my gratitude when a doctor finally verified the worm. Desdemona really had fucked someone else. It was a relief. Dr. Imaeda pulled it out and gave it to me in a jar. The maggot was the size of a fingernail clipping and the color of dirty snow, covered with tiny black teeth that looked like fuzz. The two gratifications were simultaneous: the worm was gone and I'd been right about it. I had about thirty minutes of peace before I started suspecting there might be another one left behind.

I spent the next few weeks obsessed with the open wound on my ankle, where Imaeda had cut out my maggot, looking for signs of a remaining worm in hiding. I turned from a parasite host—an actual, physical, literal host—into another kind of host: a woman with an idea, a woman who couldn't be convinced otherwise. I made my boyfriend set up "the Vaseline test" with me each night, a technique we'd found online: placing a cap full of Vaseline over the wound so the suffocated worm, this hypothetical second worm, would have no choice but to surface for air once the cap was removed.

No worm emerged, but I didn't give up looking. Maybe the worm was tricky. It had seen what happened to its comrade. I inspected the

wound relentlessly for signs of eggs or motion. Anything I found—
a stray bit of Band-Aid, a glossy patch of bruised skin or scab—was
proof. The idea of the worm—the possibility of the worm—was so
much worse than actually having a worm, because I could never get
it out. There was no *not-worm* to see, only a worm I never saw.

At the conference, when I hear that Morgellons patients often
spend hours with handheld microscopes, inspecting their own skin,
I think, *I get that.* I probably spent hours poring over my maggot
wound, its ragged edges and possible traces of parasitic life. I found
stray bits of hardened skin and weird threads—from bandages or
who-knows-what?—and I read them like tea leaves to discern what
made me feel so trapped in my own body.

I don't offer my parasite story as decisive fable. Morgellons patients aren't necessarily like the version of me who had a worm or
like the version of me who didn't. I honestly don't know what causes
the pain they feel: the rustling on their skin, their lesions, the endless threads they find emerging. I only know what I learned from
my botfly and its ghost: it was worse when I didn't have the worm
than when I did.

It's easy to forget how Sir Thomas Browne insists upon the value
of those "harsh hairs" covering the backs of his Languedoc ur-
chins. He suggests that these strange growths take off the "Unquiet
Symptoms of the Disease," "delivering" these children from their
ailments. Which is to say: physical symptoms can offer some relief.
They certainly offer tangible signs that lend themselves to diagnosis; and diagnosis can lend itself to closure.

The Morgellons diagnosis replaces one unquiet, lack of category,
with another: lack of cure. Morgellons offers an explanation, a container, and a community. It can be so difficult to admit what satis-
factions certain difficulties provide—not satisfaction in the sense
of feeling good, or being pleasurable, but in granting some shape or
substance to a discontent that might otherwise feel endless.

The trouble ends up feeling endless either way, of course—

whether it's got a vessel or not. Rita says Morgellons has taken over her whole life; she divides her life into before and after.

Kendra is one of the folks who called Rita's hotline thinking she might be crazy. Now she's here at the conference. She sits on the church steps and smokes a cigarette. She says she probably shouldn't be smoking—gesturing at the church, and then at her scarred face—but she's doing it anyway. Her chin and cheeks show sores covered with pancake makeup. But she's pretty and young, with long dark hair and a purple wide-necked shirt that makes her look like she's headed somewhere else—a day at the pool, maybe—not back into a dim Baptist church to talk about what's living under her skin.

She says the scientific presentations have all gone over her head, but she's looking forward to tomorrow's program: an interactive session with a high-magnification microscope. That's why she came all this way. She's seen things—what she mistook for hairs, and now thinks are fibers—but the microscope will see more. She'll get proof. She can't get it anywhere else. She doesn't have medical insurance and doctors don't believe her anyway. Second opinions run about half-a-month's rent. She's sick of trying to figure this out by herself. "I've messed with a part of my chin," she confesses. "It's almost like trying to pull out a piece of glass." Her chin looks like something raw and reddish has been chalked with beige powder.

Kendra makes a point of telling me she never had acne as a teenager. She wasn't one of the facially marred until she suddenly was. Now she's among others like her. She's glad to be here. It helps, she says, to know she's not the only one. Otherwise she might start thinking she was crazy again.

Folie à deux is the clinical name for shared delusions. Morgellons patients all know the phrase—it's the name of the crime they're charged with. But if *folie à deux* is happening at the conference, it's happening more like *folie à* many, *folie en masse,* an entire Baptist church full of folks having the same nightmare.

I ask Kendra if she ever doubts herself. Maybe she's afraid of something that's not actually happening?

"It's a possibility," she nods. "But at the same time, you know, I think I've got a pretty good head on my shoulders. I don't think I've totally lost all my marbles."

She tells me that coming here has made her a little bit afraid: in two years, will she be showing up in some ER with all the skin peeled off her chin? Spitting up bugs in the shower? In twenty years, will she still find her days consumed by this disease—like they already are, only more so?

She says her symptoms seem to be progressing. "Some of these things I'm trying to get out," she pauses, "it's like they move away from me."

I hate the idea that Kendra would find, in this gathering, the inevitable map of some circle of hell she's headed toward. I try to think of people who have told me about getting better, so I can tell Kendra about them. I can't think of anyone. Kendra tells me she feels for the ones who have it worse than she does.

"Everyone who is born holds dual citizenship," Susan Sontag writes, "in the kingdom of the well and in the kingdom of the sick." Most people live in the former until they are forced to take up residence in the latter. Right now Kendra is living in both. She's not entirely subsumed by sickness yet. She tells me she's meeting a friend for sushi downtown tonight. She can still understand herself outside the context of this disease: someone who does ordinary things, looks forward to the events of an ordinary life.

Only a few minutes ago, Rita was telling me these are the only three days of the year when she doesn't feel totally alone. I wonder if Kendra is following this same path—just lagging a few years behind—toward an era when she'll live full-time in the realm of illness. She says she's been finding it harder and harder to leave her house. She's too embarrassed by her face. I tell her I don't think her face is anything to be embarrassed about. "It's harder when it's your own body," I add awkwardly. "I know that."

And I *do*. I know something about that. It's about your face, but it's also about a thousand other things: an essential feeling of flaw, maybe, or a shame about taking up space, a fear of being seen as ugly or just *seen*—too much, too closely.

Here is the one place Kendra wants to be seen. She wants to be seen up close. She wants magnification. She wants evidence. She wants certainty.

"We can't all be delusional," she says.

I nod. Nodding offers me a saving vagueness—I can agree with the emotion without promising anything else. The nod can hold agnosticism and sympathy at once.

"If this weren't happening to me," Kendra continues, "if I was just hearing this from some regular person, I would probably think they were crazy."

Somehow this makes me feel for her as much as anything—that she has the grace to imagine her way into the minds of people who won't imagine hers.

"It's not just happening to you," I say finally. She thinks I mean one thing by that word—*happening*—and I think I mean another: not necessarily fibers under skin but rather some phenomenon of mind or body, maybe both in collusion, expressing god-knows-what into this lonely world.

Before the afternoon session begins, we get a musical interlude. A young man wearing jeans and flannel—somebody's Texan nephew-in-law—performs a rockabilly song about Morgellons: *"We'll guarantee you tears and applause,"* he croons, *"just take on our cause . . ."* He fumbles over the lyrics a few times because it seems like he's only doing this as a favor to his wife's step-aunt, or something like that, but he launches bravely into each song anyway: *"Doctor, doctor won't you tell me what's the matter with me / I got things going wild in my body, can't you see . . ."* The songs are part battle cry, part rain dance, part punchline, part lament.

The star of the afternoon session is a physician from Laurieton known casually around the conference as "The Australian." His talk is responding directly to the CDC report, which he calls a "load of hogwash" and a "rocking horse dung pile." He emerges as a kind of swashbuckling Aussie alligator wrestler, pinning this disease to the ground—pulling out his pidgin jujitsu to contrast the good guys (doctors who listen) with the bad guys (doctors who don't). The Australian makes it clear: He listens. He is one of the good.

He shoots to please, to get the crowd fired up, and he succeeds. He offers himself to the room as a fighter. He's talking to the margins and offering these margins the lyrics to an underdog anthem: *Doctor, doctor won't you tell me what's the matter with me* . . . He coins a new piece of jargon: DOD. Which means Delusions of Doctors. This gets applause and a few hoots from the back. The delusion? Of grandeur. The gist? That maybe *delusions of parasitosis* is just a symptom of another delusion: the hubris of thinking you know people's bodies better than they do. The Australian deploys refrain as heckling: the word *delusion* captured and lobbed back at the ones who hurled it first.

The Australian might be an egomaniac or a savior, probably both; but what matters more to me is the collective nerve he hits and the applause he gets, the specter he summons—of countless fruitless visits to countless callous doctors. One senses a hundred identical wounds across this room. Not just pocked legs and skin ribbed with the pale tracks of scars, but also smirks and muttered remarks, hastily scribbled notes, cutting gazes seeing a category, an absurdity, where a person had once been. I'm less moved by the mudslinging and more moved by the once-mud-slung-at, the ones who are clapping, and the sense of liberation underneath their applause. Here at Westoak Baptist, the Morgies get to be people once again.

Results

This isn't an essay about whether or not Morgellons disease is real. That's probably obvious by now. It's an essay about what kinds of reality are considered prerequisites for compassion. It's about this strange sympathetic limbo: Is it wrong to call it empathy when you trust the fact of suffering, but not the source? How do I inhabit someone's pain without inhabiting their particular understanding of that pain? That anxiety is embedded in every layer of this essay; even its language—every verb choice, every qualifier. Do people have parasites or claim to have them? Do they *understand* or *believe* themselves to have them? I wish I could invent a verb tense full of open spaces—a tense that didn't pretend to understand the precise mechanisms of which it spoke; a tense that could admit its own limits. As it is, I can't move an inch, finish a sentence, without running into some crisis of imputation or connotation. Every twist of syntax is an assertion of doubt or reality.

Reality means something different to everyone here. Calling Morgellons "real" generally means acknowledging there is actual, inexplicable stuff coming up through human skin whose emergence can't be explained. "Real" means fungus, parasite, bacteria, or virus, some agent causing lesions and sensations, the production of "coffee specks" of dark grain, crystalline fragments, threads, fibers, strings. In an online testimony, one woman calls her arm a sculpture garden. The trouble is that the reality of this garden—in terms of medical diagnosis, at least—depends upon doctors seeing her sculptures as well.

I find that most people at the conference understand the disease as an "us versus them" of some kind—"us" meaning patients, aligned against either the "them" of the disease itself, its parasitic agency, or else the "them" of those doctors who don't believe in it.

The notion that Morgellons patients might be "making it up" is more complicated than it seems. It could mean anything from intentional fabrication to an itch that's gotten out of hand. Itching is powerful: the impulse that tells someone to scratch lights up the same neural pathways as chemical addiction. In a *New Yorker* article titled "The Itch"—like a creature out of sci-fi—Atul Gawande tells the story of a Massachusetts woman with a chronic scalp itch who eventually scratched right into her own brain, and a man who killed himself in the night by scratching into his carotid artery. There was no discernible condition underneath their itches; no way to determine if these itches had begun on their skin or in their minds. It's not clear that itches can even be parsed in these terms. Itching that starts in the mind feels just like itching on the skin—no less real, no more fabricated—and it can begin with something as simple as a thought. It can begin with reading a paragraph like this one. Itching is a feedback loop that testifies to the possibility of symptoms that dwell in a charged and uneasy space between body and mind.

I've come to understand that the distinction made here between "real" and "unreal" doesn't just signify physical versus mental but also implies another binary: the difference between suffering produced by a force outside the self or within it. That's why "self-excoriation" is such a taboo phrase at the conference, and why patients are so deeply offended by any accusation that they've planted fibers on their own skin. These explanations place blame back on the patient and suggest not only that the harm inflicted is less legitimate but also that it's less deserving of compassion or aid. Parasites and bacteria are agents of otherness; easily granted volition as some sinister *they* or *them*, and—in holding this power—they restore the self to a victimized state.

The insistence upon an external agent of damage implies an imagining of the self as a unified entity, a collection of physical, mental, spiritual components all serving the good of some Gestalt whole— the being itself. When really, the self—at least, as I've experienced mine—is much more discordant and self-sabotaging, neither fully integrated nor consistently serving its own good.

During one discussion of possible bacterial causes for Morgellons, a woman raises her hand to make a point that seems incongruous. "Maybe there *are* no autoimmune diseases," she says; "they just don't make sense." Her point: why would a body fight itself? Perhaps, she suggests, what seems like an autoimmune disorder is simply the body anticipating a foreign invader that hasn't yet arrived. This makes sense in a way that self-destruction doesn't. Her logic is predicated on the same vision of the self as a united whole.

Ironically enough, this insistence upon a unified self seems to testify inadvertently to its inverse, a sense of the self rising up in revolt. The insistence codes as an attempt to dispel a lurking sense of the body's treachery, a sense of sickness as mutiny. The disease must be turned into an *other* so that it can be properly battled.

What does it look like when the self fights itself? When a person is broken into warring factions? Maybe it looks like the cures I see here; scraping or freezing the skin, hitting it with acid or lasers or electricity, scratching the itch or abrading it, taking cocktails of antiparasitic medicines meant for animals three times our size. All these strategies strike me as symptoms of an individual cleaved into conflicting pieces.

The abiding American myth of the self-made man comes attached to another article of faith—an insistence, even—that every self-made man can sustain whatever self he has managed to make. A man divided—thwarting or interrupting his own mechanisms of survival—fails to sustain this myth, disrupts our belief in the absolute efficacy of willpower, and in these failures also forfeits his right to our sympathy. Or so the logic goes. But I wonder why this fractured self shouldn't warrant our compassion just as much as the self besieged? Or maybe even more?

I duck out of the second afternoon session and fall into conversation with two men already involved in a tense exchange near the cookie tray. Paul is a blond Texan wearing a silver-studded belt and stiff jeans. Lenny is from Oklahoma, a well-coiffed man with a curled mustache and a dark tan. Both men wear flannel shirts tucked into their pants.

Paul is a patient, but Lenny's not. Lenny's here because he thinks he may have found the cure. A woman came to him with the disease all over her knuckles and he treated it with a laser.

I ask him to rewind: he's a dermatologist?

"Oh no!" he says. "I'm an electrician."

Who knows what kind of lasers he used? *Turned it on that,* he says; the way you'd train a gun on prey. "I turned it on that," he says, "and it killed it."

It killed *it.* The deictics are so vague. Nobody really knows what hurts or what helps. So much uncertainty is sheltered under the broad umbrella of pursuit.

This woman had two years of pain, Lenny says, and nothing helped her until he did. About twenty minutes into the conversation, he also mentions she was a meth addict. He assures us that his laser cleaned her out until there was "no sign left" of any fibers. Lenny mentions something about eggs. "They said you can look underneath where they've been. They'll lay eggs and reappear again." He says there were no eggs when he was done.

Paul has a strange look on his face as Lenny describes the cure. It seems he doesn't like the sound of it. "You didn't heal her," he says finally. "It's a virus."

Lenny nods but he's clearly taken aback. He wasn't expecting resistance.

"I've been dealing with this for eight years," Paul continues, "and I would've chopped off my hand, if that would have stopped it from spreading to the rest of my body."

You get the sense—and I don't mean this is a rhetorical or dramatic sense, but a very literal one—that he still might.

If he'd thought a laser would work, Paul continues, he would've used one. "But," he says, "I know it's more than that."

Paul looks worse than anyone else I've seen. He's been sick for eight years but only diagnosed himself with Morgellons a year ago. Before that, he had his own name for his illness: the devil's fishing bait. He says he got it on a fishing trip. Sometimes he refers to it as a virus, other times as a parasitic infestation—but the sense of sinister agency remains the same.

Paul's disease is different because you can see it. You can see it a little bit on everyone: an archipelago of scabs on a scalp; caked makeup over sores across a chin; blanched spots on tan calves. But Paul looks damaged in a different way and to a different degree. His right ear is the most obvious. It's a little twisted, a little curled, almost mashed, and it has the smooth, shiny texture of scar tissue all along the juncture between ear and jaw. I realize his mangled ear is probably something Paul did to himself, trying to get something out. *Devil's bait.* He was lured into response, into attack. His face is dotted with red pockmarks; the skin is stained with milky patterns. He's got drop-shaped scars around his eyes like he cried them.

Paul says he came home from that first fateful fishing trip with legs covered in chigger bites. "You could feel the heat coming out of my pants," he says. His whole body was inflamed.

I ask about his symptoms now. He simply shakes his head. "You can never tell what's coming next." Some days, he says, he just lies on the couch and doesn't want to see tomorrow.

I ask whether he gets support from anyone in his life. He does, he says. That's when he tells me about his sister.

At first, she wasn't sympathetic. She assumed he was on drugs when he first told her about his symptoms. But she was the one who eventually discovered Morgellons online and told him about it.

"So she's become a source of support?" I ask.

"Well," he says. "Now she has it too."

They experiment with different cures and compare notes: freezing, insecticides, dewormers for cattle, horses, dogs. A liquid nitrogen compound he injected into his ear. Lately, he says, he's had success with root beer. He pours it over his head, down his face, down his limbs.

He tells me about arriving at the ER one night with blood gushing out of his ear, screaming because he could feel them—*them* again—tearing him up inside. He tells me the doctors told him he was crazy. I tell him nothing. All I want is to look at him a different way than the doctors did that day, to make him feel a different way than they made him feel. One of those ER doctors did a physical examination and noted that his mouth was dry. Paul told them he already knew that. It was hoarse from screaming at them for help.

Paul says he probably spends ten or twelve hours a day just keeping *them* at bay, meaning whatever is inside of him. His voice is full of wariness and fear. *They* lie beyond science or significance, their ceaseless motion.

Paul doesn't seem overly impressed with the conference. Mainly because it hasn't offered a cure, he says, though there's a trace of satisfaction in his disappointment, as if certain suspicions—about futility, impossibility—have been confirmed.

Lenny jumps in again about the laser. Paul's expression verges on annoyance. Perhaps the possibility of an easy fix reduces his own vexed life to a sort of gratuitous Sisyphean labor. A cure doesn't offer hope so much as it discredits the work he's already done—exhausting every possible option, proving each one ineffectual.

Lenny seems oblivious to this. "I'm so sincere," he says. "I'm only saying, 'this is what we did, and it cured her.'" He is having a hard time thinking that his news—the news of his laser—could come across as anything but good.

I sit behind Paul through the day's final presentation. I can see he isn't paying attention to the speaker. He's looking at photographs on his computer. They're all of him—his face—mostly in profile, focused on his ear. He shows them to the middle-aged woman sitting beside him. He points to a photo of some metal implement that looks like a pair of tongs: a taser. A few moments later, I hear him whisper, "These were all eggs."

He eventually scoots his chair away from the woman and returns to what he's probably already spent days inspecting: the spectacle of his own body splayed across the screen, parsed into a thousand tiny frames of scarred and bleeding skin. It's a time-lapse arc of disfigurement. Even here, among others who identify with the same malady, he retreats into the terrible privacy of his own broken body. He brings others—strangers, briefly—into this quiet battleground, but it's always just him again, eventually, drawn back into the cloister of his damage, that nearly unfathomable loneliness.

When I leave the church, I find sunlight waiting outside our windowless rooms. The world has been patient. Springtime in Austin is grackles in the trees; a nearly invisible fluttering of bats under the Congress Avenue bridge, a flickering of wings and waft of guano in blue-washed twilight. Austin is beautiful women everywhere, in scarves and sunglasses; BBQ smoke rising into thick sunlight; wind-blown oak leaves skittering across patios where I eat oysters on ice. Austin is throw-a-stone-and-you-hit-a-food-truck, each one gourmet, serving tongue-on-rice, fried avocado tacos, donuts topped with bacon. Dusk holds the clicking metronome of cowboy boots on sidewalks. People with narrative tattoos smoke in the heat. I find a grotto dedicated to the Virgin Mary with an empty beer bottle and a bag of Cheez-Its buried in the gravel.

I walk among the young and healthy and I am more or less one of them. I am trying not to itch. I am trying not to think about whether I'm itching. I am trying not to take my skin for granted. Sometimes my heart beats too fast, or a worm lodges under the skin of my ankle, or I drink too much, or I am too thin, but these are sojourns away from a kingdom I can generally claim—of being *okay*, capable of desire and being desired, full of a sense I belong in the world. But when I leave the Baptist church on Slaughter Lane, I can't quiet the voices of those who no longer feel they belong anywhere. I spend a day in their kingdom and then leave when I please. It feels like a betrayal to come up for air.

Doubting Morgellons hasn't stopped me from being afraid I'll get it. I buffered myself before the conference: "If I come back from Austin thinking I have Morgellons," I told my friends, "you have to tell me I don't have Morgellons." Now that I'm here, I wash my hands a lot. I'm conscious of other people's bodies.

Then it starts happening, as I knew it would. After a shower, I notice small blue strands curled like tiny worms across my clavicle. I find what appear to be minuscule spines, little quills, tucked into the crevice of a fortune line on my palm. I've got these fleeting moments of catching sight, catching panic. I'm afraid to submit myself to the public microscope inspection because I'm nervous something will be found and I won't be able to let go of it.

It actually gives me an odd thrill. Maybe some part of me *wants* to find something. I could be my own proof. Or else I could write a first-person story about delusion. I could connect to the disease with filaments of my own, real or imagined, under my skin.

If you look closely enough, of course, skin is always foreign, anyone's—full of strange bumps, botched hairs, hefty freckles, odd patches of flush and rough. The blue fibers are probably just stray threads from a towel, or from my sleeve, the quills not quills at all but just smeared pen ink. But it's in these moments of fear, oddly, that I come closest to experiencing Morgellons the way its patients do: its symptoms physical and sinister, its tactics utterly invasive. Inhabiting their perspective only makes me want to protect myself from what they have. I wonder if these are the only options available to my crippled organs of compassion: I'm either full of disbelief, or else I'm washing my hands in the bathroom.

I'm not the only person at the conference thinking about contagion. One woman stands up to say she needs to know the facts about how Morgellons is really transmitted. She tells the crowd that her family and friends refuse to come to her apartment. She needs proof they can't catch the disease from her couch. It's hard not to speculate. Her family might be afraid of catching her disease, but they might be even more afraid there's nothing to catch; maybe they're keeping their distance from her obsession instead. I hear so much sadness in what she says—*tell me it's not contagious, so everyone will come back*—and so much hope for an answer that might make things better; that might make her less alone.

Kendra tells me she's afraid of getting her friends sick whenever she goes out to dinner with them. I picture her eating sushi downtown—handling her chopsticks so carefully, keeping her wasabi under strict quarantine—so that this *thing* in her—this thing with agency, if not category—won't get into anyone else. Her fear underscores an unspoken tension embedded in the premise of the conference itself: the notion that all these folks with a possibly contagious condition might gather together in the same confined space.

The specter of contagion actually serves a curious double function. On the one hand, as with Kendra, there is the shameful sense of oneself as a potential carrier of infection. But on the other hand

the possibility of spreading this disease also suggests that it's real—
that it could be proven by its manifestation in others.

One of the strangest corners of the Morgellons online labyrinth—a
complicated network of chat boards, personal testimonies, and
high-magnification photographs—is the "Pets of Morgellons" website. I realize quickly that it's neither a joke nor a feel-good photo
album. It's not just "pets of [people who have] Morgellons" but "pets
[who also have] Morgellons." In a typical entry, a cat named Ika introduces herself and her illness:

> I have been named [for] the Japanese snack of dried cuttlefish . . .
> Typically I am full of chaotic energy, however lately I have
> been feeling quite lethargic and VERY itchy. My best friend /
> mommy thinks that she gave me her skin condition, and she is so
> very SAD. I think she is even more sad that she passed it on to
> me than the fact that she has it covering her entire face.

The list continues, a litany of sick animals: a sleek white dog
named Jazzy sports itchy paws; two bloodhounds are biting invisible fleas; a Lhasa apso joins his mother for stretches in an infrared
sauna. One entry is an elegy for an Akita named Sinbad:

> It appears that I got the disease at the same time that my beau-
> tiful lady owner got it. And after many trips to the vet they
> had to put me down. I know it was for my own good, but I do
> miss them a lot. I can still see my master's face, right up close to
> mine, when the doc put me to sleep . . . I could sniff his breath
> and feel the pain in his eyes as tears rolled down his face. But,
> it's ok. I'm alright now. The maddening itching is finally over.
> I'm finally at peace.

The ending paints resolution over pathos. We read, *I'm finally
at peace*, and imagine another who probably isn't: the master who
cried when he put his dog to sleep. Who knows what happened to

Sinbad? Maybe he really did need to get put down; maybe he was old, or sick with something else. Maybe he wasn't sick at all. But he has become part of an illness narrative—like lesions, or divorces, or the fibers themselves. He is irrefutable proof that suffering has happened, that things have been lost.

The second day of the conference kicks off with a Japanese television documentary about Morgellons. Over there they call it "cotton erupting disease," suggesting a stage prank—a great *poof!*—more than the silent sinister curling of microscopic fibers. The program has been loosely translated. We see a woman standing at her kitchen counter, mixing a livestock antiparasitic called Ivermectin into a glass of water. The Japanese voiceover sounds concerned and the English translator fills in: she knows this antiparasitic isn't for human consumption, but she's using it anyway. She's desperate. We see a map of America with patches of known cases breaking out like lesions over the land, a twisted Manifest Destiny: disease claims community, claims the disordered as kin. Just as fibers attach to an open wound—its wet surface a kind of glue—so does the notion of disease function as an adhesive, gathering anything we can't understand, anything that hurts, anything that will stick. *Transmission by Internet*, some skeptics claim about Morgellons—chat boards as pied pipers, calling all comers. It's true that Morgellons wasn't officially born until 2001. It's grown up alongside the Internet. Its online community has become an authority in its own right. People here don't necessarily agree about the particulars of their shared disease—bacteria, fungus, parasite—but they agree about a feeling of inescapability: wherever you go, the disease follows; whatever you do, it resists.

A woman named Sandra pulls out her cell phone to show me a photo of something she coughed up. It looks like a little albino shrimp. She thinks it's a larva. She photographed it through a jeweler's loupe. She wants a microscope but doesn't have one yet. She put the larva on a book to give a sense of scale. I try to get a good look at the print; I'm curious about what she was reading. My mind seeks the quiet hours—how this woman fills her life beyond the condition of infestation, as that *beyond* keeps getting smaller.

Sandra has a theory about the fibers—not that the fibers *are* an organism but that the organisms inside her are gathering these fibers to make their cocoons. This explains why so many of the fibers turn out to be ordinary kinds of thread, dog hairs or cotton fibers. Their danger is one of purpose, not of kind: creatures making a nest of her body, using the ordinary materials of her life to build a home inside of her.

Once I've squinted long enough at the shrimpish thing, Sandra brings up a video of herself in the bathtub. "These are way beyond fibers," she promises. Only her feet are visible protruding through the surface of the water. The quality is grainy, but it appears the bath is full of wriggling larva. Their forms are hard to feel sure about—everything is dim and a little sludgy—but that's actually what it looks like. She says that a couple years ago there were hundreds coming out of her skin. It's gotten a little better. When she takes a bath, only two or three of those worms come out.

I'm really at a loss. I don't know if what I'm seeing are worms, or where they come from, or what they might be if they're *not* worms, or whether I want them to be worms or not, or what I have to believe about this woman if they aren't worms, or about the world or human bodies or this disease if they *are*. But I do know I see a bunch of little wriggling shadows, and for now I'm glad I'm not a doctor or a scientist or basically anyone who knows anything about anything, because this uncertainty lets me believe Sandra without needing to confirm her. I can dwell with her—for just a moment, at least—in the possibility of those worms, in that horror. She's been alone in it for so long.

I catch sight of Kendra watching Sandra's cell phone. She's wondering if this is what her future holds. I tell her that everyone's disease turns out a little different. But what do I know? Maybe her future looks like this too.

Kendra tells me about sushi last night. It was good. She had fun. She actually ended up buying a painting from the restaurant. She shouldn't have, she says. She doesn't have the money. But she saw it hanging on the wall and couldn't resist. She shows me a cell phone picture: lush braided swirls of oil paint curl from the corners of a parchment-colored square. The braids are jewel toned, deeply saturated, royal purple twined with lavender and turquoise.

I think but don't say: *fibers.*

"You know," she says, voice lowered. "It reminds me a little of those things."

I get a sinking feeling. It's that moment in an epidemic movie when the illness spreads beyond its quarantine. Even when Kendra leaves this kingdom of the sick, she finds sickness waiting patiently for her on the other side. She pays three hundred dollars she can't afford just so she can take its portrait home with her. Whatever comfort I took in her sushi outing, it's gone now. Like I said, disease gathers anything that will stick. Even art on restaurant walls starts to look like what's wrong with you, even if you can't see it—can't see, but see everywhere.

During the morning program, the conference organizers pass around a sheet of jokes—"You might be a morgie if"—followed by a list of punchlines: "You scratch more than the dog," "You've been fired by more doctors than bosses," "An acid bath and total body shave sounds like a fun Friday night." Some jokes summon the split between the current self and the self before its disease: "past life regression means remembering any time before Morgellons." Others summon the split between the self and others: "at dinner your family uses oil and vinegar on their salads while you dump them on your hair and body." Some of the jokes I don't even get: "You can't use anything on your computer that requires a USB port because there's NO WAY you're disconnecting your QX-3 Digital Blue."

I look up QX-3 Digital Blue: it's a microscope. The website claims you can use it to "satisfy your basic curiosity of the world around you," which makes me think of Paul's computer—his own body photographed over and over again—how small his world has gotten.

I don't see any QX-3s at the conference, but the organizers are holding a lottery to give away some less expensive microscopes: a handful of miniscopes, like small black plums, and their larger cousin the EyeClops, a children's toy. At Amazon, I find the EyeClops advertised in terms of alchemy. "Ordinary to Extraordinary," the description brags, "minuscule salt crystals morph into blocks of ice; hair and carpet turn into giant noodles; and small insects become fearsome creatures." This ad copy transforms the alchemy of Morgellons into a magic trick: examined close-up, our most ordinary parts—even the surface and abrasions of our skin—become wild and terrifying.

My name is automatically entered in the lottery, along with all the other conference attendees, and I end up winning a miniscope. I'm sheepish headed to the stage. What do I need a scope for? I'm here to write about how other people need scopes. I'm given a square box a bit smaller than a Rubik's Cube. I imagine how the scene will play out later tonight: examining my skin in the stale privacy of my hotel room, coming face to face with that razor's edge between skepticism and fear by way of the little widget in my palm.

At the bottom of my sheet of jokes, the title—*You might be a morgie if*—is given one last completing clause: "you laughed out loud and 'got' these jokes." I remember that early e-mail—*topic of the biggest joke in the world*—and see why these jokes might matter so much—not simply because they resonate, but because they reclaim the activity of joking itself. Here Morgies are the makers of jokes, not their targets. Every joke recycles the traitorous body into a neatly packaged punchline.

So we get our page of jokes and I get some of them, but not all of them, and Sandra gets an audience for her cell phone slideshow and I get a miniscope I didn't even want and Kendra gets a painting—and, in the end, she also gets the microscope consultation she's been waiting for.

Afterward, I ask her how it went. She tells me it's been confirmed: Rita found threads around her eyes. But she shrugs as she says it—as if the discovery is just an anticlimax; offering none of the resolution or solidity it promised.

"I'm fucking myself," Kendra tells me, "the more I try to pick them away."

I agree. I nod.

"The more I try to pick them away," she continues, "the more come . . . like they want to show me I can't get rid of them that easily."

Discussion

In the end, I gave my miniscope away.

I gave it to Sandra. I gave it to her because she was sick of using her jeweler's loupe, because she was sad she hadn't gotten one, and because I felt self-conscious about winning one when I wasn't even looking for fibers in the first place.

"That's so generous," she said to me when I gave it to her—and of course I'd been hoping she would say that. I wanted to do nice things for everyone out of a sense of preemptive guilt that I couldn't conceptualize this disease in the same way as those who suffered from it. So I said, *Here, take my miniscope,* in hopes that might make up for everything else.

That's so generous. But maybe it wasn't. Maybe it was just the opposite. Maybe I just took hours of her life away and replaced them with hours spent at the peephole of that microscope, staring at what she wouldn't be able to cure.

A confession: I left the conference early. I actually, embarrassingly, went to *sit by the shitty hotel pool* because I felt emotionally drained and like I deserved it. I baked bare skinned in the Texan sun and watched a woman from the conference come outside and carefully lay her own body, fully clothed, across a reclining chair in the shade.

Acknowledgments

I've left the kingdom of the ill. Dawn and Kendra and Paul and Rita remain. Now I get the sunlight and they don't. They feed themselves horse dewormers and I don't. But I still feel the ache of an

uncanny proximity. They have no fear that isn't mine, no dread of
self I haven't known. I kept telling them, *I can't imagine,* and every
once in a while, softer, *I can.*

When does empathy actually reinforce the pain it wants to console? Does giving people a space to talk about their disease—probe
it, gaze at it, share it—help them move through it, or simply deepen
its hold? Does a gathering like this offer solace or simply confirm
the cloister and prerogative of suffering? Maybe it just pushes
on the pain until it gets even worse, until it requires more comforting than it did before. The conference seems to confirm, in those
who attend, the sense that they will only ever get what they need
here. It sharpens the isolation it wants to heal.

I can only be myself when I'm here, is something I heard more
than once. But every time I left the dim rooms of Westoak Baptist,
I found myself wishing its citizens could also be themselves elsewhere, could be themselves anywhere—in the lavish Austin sun-
shine, for starters, or hunched over artisanal donuts at a picnic table
on a warm night. I wanted them to understand themselves as constituted and contoured beyond the margins of illness.

I think of how Paul always does his grocery shopping half an
hour before closing time so he won't see anyone he knows; I think
of the bald man sitting behind me on the second day, whose name I
never learned, who doesn't do much besides shuttle between a bare
apartment and an unnamed job; I think of a beautiful woman who
wonders how any man could ever love her scarred.

Kendra is terrified by the same assurances that offer her valida-
tion. She has proof of fibers in her skin but no hope of getting them
out, only a vision of what it might look like to be consumed by this
disease entirely: a thousand bloody photographs on her computer,
a soup of larvae on her cell phone testifying to the passing days of
her life.

What did Kendra say? *Some of these things I'm trying to get out,
it's like they move away from me.* Isn't that all of us? Sometimes we're
all trying to purge something. And what we're trying to purge resists our purging. *Devil's bait*—this disease offers a constant feeling

of being lured, the promise of resolution dangling just out of reach. These demons belong to all of us: an obsession with our boundaries and visible shapes, a fear of invasion or contamination, an understanding of ourselves as perpetually misunderstood.

But doesn't this search for meaning obfsucate the illness itself? It's another kind of bait, another tied-and-painted fly: the notion that if we understand something well enough, we can make it go away.

Everyone I met at the conference was kind. They offered their warmth to me and to each other. I was a visitor to what they knew, but I have been a citizen at times—a citizen subject to that bodily unrest—and I know I'll be one again. I was splitting my time between one Austin and another; I was splitting my time between dim rooms and open skies.

One of the speakers quoted nineteenth-century biologist Thomas Huxley:

> Sit down before fact as a little child, be prepared to give up every preconceived notion, follow humbly wherever and to whatever abyss Nature leads, or you shall learn nothing.

I want to sit down in front of everyone I've heard—listen to their voices in my tape recorder like a child, like an agnostic, like a pluralist. I want to be the compassionate nurse, not the skeptical doctor. I want the abyss, not the verdict. I want to believe everyone. I want everyone to be right. But compassion isn't the same thing as belief. This isn't a lesson I want to learn.

It wasn't until the seventeenth century that the words *pity* and *piety* were fully distinguished. Sympathy was understood as a kind of duty, an obligation to some basic human bond—and what I feel toward this disorder is a kind of piety. I feel an obligation to pay homage or at least accord some reverence to these patients' collective understanding of what makes them hurt. Maybe it's a kind of sympathetic infection in its own right: this need to go-along-with, to nod-along-with, to support; to agree.

Paul said, "I wouldn't tell anyone my crazy-ass symptoms." But he told them to me. He's always been met with disbelief. He called it "typical." Now I'm haunted by that word. For Paul, life has become a pattern and the moral of that pattern is, *you're destined for this.* The disbelief of others is inevitable and so is loneliness; both are just as much a part of this disease as any fiber, any speck or crystal or parasite.

I went to Austin because I wanted to be a different kind of listener than the kind these patients had known: doctors winking at their residents, friends biting their lips, skeptics smiling in smug bewilderment. But wanting to be different doesn't make you so. Paul told me his crazy-ass symptoms and I didn't believe him. Or at least, I didn't believe him the way he wanted to be believed. I didn't believe there were parasites laying thousands of eggs under his skin, but I did believe he hurt like there were. Which was typical. I was typical. In writing this essay, how am I doing something he wouldn't understand as betrayal? I want to say, *I heard you.* To say, *I pass no verdicts.* But I can't say these things to him. So instead I say this: I think he can heal. I hope he does.

✠ LA FRONTERA ✠

San Ysidro

I'm at the busiest land border in the world. I get across quickly because I'm headed in the right direction, by which I mean the wrong direction. I'm going where no one wants to stay. On the opposite side of Highway 5, a sparkling line of gridlock points north toward the United States of America.

Over there, the traffic lanes are supermarket aisles. You can buy popcorn, cookies, lollipops, cigarettes. You want coffee? You can get it from a boy barely tall enough to reach your car window. You want the paper in Spanish? Great. In English? Maybe. You want an animal-print towel? There are hundreds.

I'm headed to a literary gathering held in Tijuana and Mexicali that's been billed as an *encuentro*. I've gathered this means something between "festival" and "conference," but when I think of *encuentro* I hear the word for "story" *(cuento)* coaxed from the word for "encounter" *(encontrar)*—an intersection that hints at what will happen at this upheaval of debauchery and roundtables: Stories will be currency, people will be signing books, people will be confused, people will be making book deals, people will be talking shit about Mexicali and wishing they were in Oaxaca. People will be having sex. Nothing will happen on time. Cookies will be served with Styrofoam cups of coffee in the morning. Cocaine will be served in bathroom stalls at night.

This is 2010. I hear that Tijuana has gotten much better in the past two years, which is what the American media has recently begun to say as well. But variations and fluctuations are inevitably glossed over in conversations where we, up north, talk about how bad it's gotten "down there." Of course, *down there* isn't one place but a thousand, and the truth is it's gotten better in Tijuana and much worse in Tamaulipas and simply stayed horrible in Ciudad Juárez, where life is so violent it's hard to understand the gradations between bad and worse.

Someone tells me about living in Tijuana during the worst months—not so much about living under the constant threat of violence but about *talking* about living under constant threat of violence. It's impossible to speak, she says, when you're still in the middle of it.

This is what it was like in Tijuana, a few years back: Even when people got together for dinner, somewhere private, they wouldn't focus on what their lives had become: scared to go drinking, scared to go to work, scared to catch a bus or buy a pack of cigarettes or cross the fucking street. Now they can talk. Speaking is easier when the worst has been pushed out of earshot—past the point of being taunted, by delusions of safety, into some vengeful return.

Tijuana

Avenida Revolución is lined with the hollowed husks of cheap tourism. Empty bars stand like relics of a vanished civilization felled by its own hedonistic excess: silent dance floors framed by thatched walls and faux-jungle decor, balconies full of tiki torches and flapping banners advertising tequila happy hours no one is attending. The clubs feel like foreclosed homes. The tourists have been scared away. Some must still come, I suppose, but I don't see any of them on the streets. The Centro Cultural Tijuana has a surprisingly lovely domed ceiling fitted with squares of glass that filter the sunlight into jeweled colors: fuchsia, tangerine, deep mint. But the only people I see inside are men selling bus tickets to other places.

Everyone is hawking wares along the streets, but no one is buying. If I wanted, I could get all kinds of things: a zebra-striped burro, postcards showing ten pairs of titties and the red stump of a Tecate can in the sand, a little frog carved by an old man *before my very eyes* and fitted with an actual cigarette between its wooden lips. I could get a

T-shirt printed with the stoic face of Pancho Villa or the inevitable face of Che, a T-shirt with a joke about beer, another T-shirt with a joke about beer, a T-shirt with a joke about tequila, a T-shirt with a joke about mixing beer and tequila, or a T-shirt that gets to the heart of what all this drinking is about (this one in English: "I Fuck on the First Date"). Conveniently enough, there's a hotel across from all these kitsch bodegas that advertises rooms for ninety-nine pesos an hour. I don't see anyone going in or coming out.

The whole time I am thinking of Tijuana two years ago, the never talking. All across the border, other towns are still in the thick of this unspeaking. The people who call Ciudad Juárez the most dangerous city in the world are the ones who don't live there.

I think maybe if I walk the streets where someone was afraid, where an entire city was afraid, I'll maybe understand the fear a little better. This is the grand fiction of tourism, that bringing our bodies somewhere draws that place closer to us, or we to it. It's a quick fix of empathy. We take it like a shot of tequila, or a bump of coke from the key to a stranger's home. We want the inebriation of presence to dissolve the fact of difference. Sometimes the city fucks on the first date, and sometimes it doesn't. But always, *always*, we wake up in the morning and find we didn't know it at all.

I wake up in the morning and get *huevos con jamón* at a place called Tijuana Tilly's. I could have gotten a waffle but I didn't. I could have gotten *pan francés* with whipped cream, but I didn't. I'm going authentic. I'm eating with a publicist named Paola and a novelist named Adán. They both get waffles. Paola tells me she can't believe that DF (Mexico City) is quite possibly the safest place in Mexico these days. Not what she's used to. Adán tells me Mexicali, where we're going to meet the other writers for the conference, is relatively safe as well. *Relatively* is an important word around here.

Mexicali, in any case, is two hours east. It first exploded during Prohibition, just like Tijuana, but otherwise they're not much alike. Adán's Spanish is fast and I'm not sure if I'm getting the gist of what he's saying—or at least, the right gist—because it seems like he's talking about an underground town full of Chinese people. As it turns out, my Spanish is close. During the 1920s, Chinese laborers outnumbered Mexicans in Mexicali by a ratio of eight to one, and a network of subterranean tunnels connected their opium dens and brothels to those eager and prohibited Americans living just across the border.

Tijuana blurs. Once I leave, I'm eager to talk about it—the way you're eager to talk about a dream when you wake up, afraid it will dissolve if you don't pin the details to their places, sketch a path between absurdities. As soon as I leave it, I think, what *was* that city? It was an unlit hallway next to an office with broken windows (my hostel) and a plate of shredded pork cooked with oranges (my dinner). It was a band composed of young men called La Sonrisa Vertical (the Vertical Smile) and a band composed of old men, I don't know what they were called, who asked repeatedly for more Charles Shaw Shiraz and played the hell out of their electric guitars. They had two eggs perched on their amp, maybe raw, maybe hardboiled, not making any sense but belonging absolutely where they were.

Mexicali

If the road into Tijuana is clogged with guns and cars and men in uniform, the pageantry of American panic, the highway out is dust ravaged and ghostly, snaking from the outer barrios to the gaunt hills of a frontier desert. Beyond city limits, shacks perch on muddy slopes strewn with bits of wall and fence. Many have been wrapped or roofed in billboard posters. They look like presents. Their sides show the giant toothpaste tubes and human smiles of advertisements. Eventually, the slums give way to an infamous highway known as the Rumorosa, a roller coaster that twists and dips through the hairpin turns and rock-slide slopes of bleached red mountains.

At a lookout point halfway to Mexicali, where the road drops off raggedly to our left, we emerge around a bend to see the partially blackened wreckage of a semi-truck. The cab is inches from the edge of the cliff. A man is curled fetal on the ground, bleeding from his forehead. He doesn't look dead. There isn't an ambulance in sight, but a priest stands over the man's body, blocking him from the noon sun and muttering words of prayer, waving at the passing cars: *Slow down, slow down.* It must be ninety in October and this man wears black vestments that soak up the whole of the heat. His cross glitters silver. The grill of the truck glitters silver behind him.

It's not just that violence *happens* here—intentional, casual, accidental, incidental—it's that the prospect and the aftermath of violence are constantly crowding you from all sides: men with machine guns on the Avenida Revolución, growling dogs leaping into SUVs to sniff for drugs, a drunk passed out in front of the *panadería*, a driver so tired or tweaking he barrels his semi into a cliff. We pass a soldier standing alert with a semiautomatic in his hands, apparently guarding the giant pile of scrap tires behind him. There's nothing else in sight. The soldiers of the country stand ready against an uncontrollable violence, perched on trash, their guns pointed at thin air.

In a 2010 op-ed in the *New York Times,* Elmer Mendoza reports that when a troop of Niños Exploradores (something like Boy Scouts) was brought to welcome officials visiting Ciudad Juárez, their scoutmaster took them through a call-and-response routine. "How do the children play in Juárez?" he called. The boys all dropped to the ground.

At a drug checkpoint, our entire van is emptied out. Larger vehicles inevitably attract more suspicion. The soldiers empty our bags. It all feels pro forma, but still—of a climate, of a piece, setting a tone. As we drive away, I glance back and notice that another soldier, this one standing on a truck, had his machine gun trained on us the whole time.

There are no flashy clubs in Mexicali, no zebra burros, no drink specials. You couldn't find a smoking frog to save your life. You can get plastic bags full of chopped cactus or cigarettes for cheap. The closest thing to a Spanglish shot glass is the sound track at a club called SlowTime, where a woman's voice moans over and over again: "Oh, you fucking me makes me bilingual."

The light is harsher in this city, everything dustier. The hotels advertise rates for four hours instead of one. I don't know what this means, but it seems to mark an important difference in civic culture.

Chinatown is alive and well aboveground. Restaurants serve bean curd with salsa and shark-fin tacos. I eat lunch at Dragón de Oro, whose parking lot runs up against the border itself, a thick brown fence about twenty feet high. The stucco homes and baseball diamonds of Calexico are barely visible through the slats.

We are fifty strong, we *encuentro*-goers. There's Oscar, a poet who tells me his vision of Heidegger over chilaquiles one morning, and Kelly, a simultaneous interpreter who is writing a Spanish glossary of erotic language. There's Marco, another poet, who walks across the border to buy a new pair of Converse in Calexico. Marco informs me that he abandoned his "lyric self" about a year ago, once his city grew so violent he got scared to leave his house. He needs a new poetry these days. He's interested in repurposing in general and Flarf in particular—an experimental poetic practice that involves sorting and distilling the vast innards of the Internet, whittling by way of search term, juxtaposing odd results, often to the point of absurdity, hilarity. Marco believes in hilarity. Marco teaches college students. His life sounds a lot like mine until it absolutely doesn't. The night before coming to Mexicali, he stayed up till one thirty to finish grading a batch of papers, then decided to reward himself the next morning by hitting the snooze button. Fair enough. As it turned out, a grenade explosion woke him anyway, two minutes later, followed by a volley of machine-gun fire. "Like a conversation," he says, "one voice and then the response." He says it wasn't anything unusual.

I meet the founder of something called the Shandy Conspiracy. Every time he sees me, he asks if I'm ready to be Shandyized. All I know about this process is that it will involve subtlety and darkness. He puts out a magazine (the epicenter of his conspiracy) whose masthead features a lion attacking a zebra. Instead of blood, the zebra's neck issues jets of rainbow fluid. It's Darwin on acid. I catch myself looking at all the artwork here in terms of sociopolitical fractals: How can I see the narco war contained in every illustrated zebra? It's a strange feeling, watching quirk spew from the jaws of war—like a guttural cry, flayed and searing, this absurd fountain of rainbow blood. I bend everything according to the gravity of conflict.

More accurately put, I bend what I can understand. There's so much that eludes me. In a crowd of bilingual writers, my Spanish is embarrassing, and this embarrassment starts to shade into a deeper sense of political and national shame. I'm afraid to talk about the current landscape of the narco wars because I'm afraid of getting something wrong. Americans are known for getting things wrong when it comes to conflicts in other countries. So I listen. I gradually get a sense of the terrain. The Sinaloa Cartel controls much of the Western Seaboard—where most of the weed is grown, and a frontier mythos maintains the drug dealer as outlaw—while the Gulf Cartel operates along the Gulf, trafficking coke and Central American illegals called *pollos*, peasants whom they either smuggle or extort.

Reading about the drug wars is like untangling a web of intricate double negatives. One cartel pays a prison warden to set prisoners free at night so they can act as assassins targeting the key players in another cartel, then the targeted cartel captures a police officer and tortures him until he admits to this corruption. They tape and broadcast his confession. The authorities step in, the warden is removed, the prisoners riot to bring her back; the reporters who cover the riots are kidnapped by the rivals of the cartel that released the videotape of the tortured officer. They counter-release their own videotapes of other tortured men confessing to other corruptions. Got it?

Tracking the particulars is like listening to a horrific kind of witty banter in a language built for others' mouths, finding yourself participating in a conversation in which you have no ability to speak. "Conversation" means something new in this place: a flood of words I can't understand, the call-and-response patter of semiautomatics I've never heard.

I get to know another cast, not authors but killers: There's El Teo, vying for control of the Tijuana Cartel, who likes to kill at parties because it makes his message more visible; and there's El Pozolero ("the Stewmaker"), who dissolves El Teo's victims in acid once their message needs to turn invisible again. The most famous drug lord in Mexico is El Chapo ("Shorty"), head of the Sinaloa Cartel and currently ranked sixtieth on *Forbes's* list of the most powerful people in the world. That puts him behind Barack Obama (2), Osama bin Laden (57), and the Dalai Lama (39), but ahead of Oprah Winfrey (64) and Julian Assange (68). The president of Mexico didn't make the list at all. In Mexicali, I find myself learning the statistics of two economies—authors don't get paid advances for their work, hit men in Ciudad Juárez get two thousand pesos a job—and the contours of two parallel geographies, one mapping the narco wars and another the landscape of literary production. This first topography is tissued like a horrible veil across the second. Durango, for example, is where El Chapo found his teenage bride, but it's also home to a poet who wears combat boots and spits when he reads his poems, which are mostly about tits. Sinaloa is home to its namesake cartel, but it's also home to Oscar and his Heidegger study groups. The capital of Sinaloa, Culiacán, has a cemetery full of two-story drug-lord mausoleums, impeccably furnished and air-conditioned for the comfort of mourning friends and family. Across town from these palaces, Oscar lives in a house with his kitten, Heidie. I imagine an entire menagerie: a dog named Dasein, two birds named Tiempo and Ser. I imagine an air conditioner humming quietly next to the ashes of a man. I am trying to merge these two Sinaloas, to make them the same.

The geography lesson moves east: Tamaulipas is a region famous for the August massacre of seventy-two illegals who wouldn't pay up when the Cártel del Golfo asked them to. *Wouldn't.* Right. Couldn't. But Tamaulipas is also home to Marco, the poet interested in Flarf. When I think of Flarf, I think of poems that deconstruct and splice together blog posts about Iraqi oil and Justin Timberlake's sex life. It's true that Marco is up to something like this, but his project is made of different materials and perhaps a bit less irony. He is repurposing the language of the conflict for his poems. He trolls Internet message boards full of posts from people sequestered in their homes. He takes phrases from the signs that cartels leave on the corpses of their victims, and scraps from the messages they scribble onto the skin of the dead. He cuts up quotes; fits the puzzle pieces of fear back together to make his poems. This is a new iteration: Flarf *from* and *for* and *of* the narco wars. Narco-Flarf. I wonder how this kind of work preserves that part of Flarf that feels so central: its sense of humor. I wonder whether this matters. To judge from how often Marco laughs (very), it matters a lot.

The whole *encuentro* is an odd mixture of revelry and seriousness. People speak constantly and painfully about the narco wars but they also do a lot of coke. They do it off one another's house keys, just like I imagined they would, and I find myself wondering about those keys and the locks they turn. How many locks do people have in their homes? More than they did before? How often do they go to sleep afraid?

Just a few weeks before coming to Mexicali, Marco presented his work at a Los Angeles gallery called LACE. He named his piece *SPAM*. It was a wall hanging that showcased a poem he'd made from message-board fragments—in this case, posts from residents of Comales, a barrio on the outskirts of Tamaulipas that had essentially become a cluster of hideout bunkers.

Marco called the neighborhood *zona cero*. Ground zero.

On the Internet, and in Marco's work, these *zona cero* voices find a mobility their bodies have been denied: *"no se trabaja, no hay escuela, tiendas cerradas . . . estamos muriendo poco a poco"* ("there isn't work, there isn't school, the shops are closed . . . we are dying little by little"). The language isn't "poetic" because it didn't start as poetry. It started as a cry. And now it's something else. Marco, of course, abandoned his lyric self last year. Now his poems have no single speaker but a mass of ordinary voices that speak these desperate words, coaxed into cadence by his own sequestered hands.

SPAM was made in Tamaulipas and shown in Los Angeles, but it's composed of materials from an immaterial network (the

Internet) that hangs suspended, contrapuntal and infinite, in between these places and essentially in no place at all. The piece has some faith in the Internet but also understands how it abstracts experience into something nonsensical or illegible (spam!). The piece mocks borders but speaks explicitly toward them: "*La pieza intentará crear diálogo más allá de las fronteras . . .*" The piece is not simply a dispatch, Marco writes, but rather part of a conversation—the same conversation, I can't help thinking, as the grenade explosion on his street.

Calexico

It's right *there*, Calexico, just past the brown fence. You can see recycling bins overturned on its asphalt driveways. But it takes more than an hour to cross the border. And this is four thirty in the morning, when we go, and this isn't even Tijuana. San Ysidro can take five hours if you hit it at the wrong time.

For some Mexicans, the border isn't a big deal. Some lucky few get the border's equivalent of a freeway E-ZPass. Marco thinks nothing of crossing here for a new pair of sneakers, though he shies away from crossing near home because the border is more dangerous in Golfo territory.

For others, the *frontera* is the edge of the world. Manuel, a keyboardist, explains that he'd love to play a gig in California but knows he never will. He can't even spare the money for the phone call to make the appointment for the visa interview, much less sport a bank account flush enough to get one.

I cross from Mexicali with Marco and a Peruvian novelist. We're driving a dusty red Jeep. Our variety pack of nationalities sets the officer on edge. He doesn't seem reassured by our explanation. An *encuentro?* Interesting. He gives me a hard time. This is also interesting. I've returned to America from many foreign countries. I've never been given a hard time. I'm always profiled, and it always works to my advantage. Now I'm with company. I've forgotten to remove a yellow-fever vaccination certificate from my passport, and apparently this is a problem. The border officer shoves the paper in my face. "What's this?" he says. "You have a dog?" I don't know what he's talking about, but I don't have a dog and I tell him so. "But you're from the States?" he says, as if I've contradicted myself. I tell him I am, but I can hear something strange: the inflection of a question trilling faintly through my voice, as if I'm no longer sure. Perhaps I've done something wrong. Marco explains: "They try to trip you up."

The truth doesn't necessarily serve you too well, either. Let's say you're an old Mexican woman with grown children who live in the United States. You'd better not mention them at your visa interview. You might think they'd be a reason to grant you entry, but really they're the best possible reason to keep you out. This woman was real, Marco tells me. He stood behind her in the consulate line. There are probably six of her, ten of her, a thousand of her all across the border. As they say: *she actually happened.* She'd already been denied three times, kept paying a hundred dollars to apply again, kept talking about her kids, was running out of cheeks to turn, was running out of money.

Calexico is a small town with an ugly main drag full of *casas de cambio* (currency exchanges), but the fields on the outskirts of town are lush and emerald in the dawn. Everything around Mexicali was dry, dry, dry. "The grass is always greener," says Marco, and I laugh. Is this all right, that I'm laughing? I think so.

We pass an interior immigration station, a second layer of defense constructed in lieu of designing any kind of decent immigration policy. It flaunts its statistics like the scoreboard at a sporting event: 3,567 immigration arrests, 370 criminal arrests, 9,952 pounds of drugs seized. Marco asks, What do these numbers *mean?* There are no dates. The figures are simply toys, emptied of context and significance. Presumably, the stats are meant to scare illiterate *pollos* by osmosis or maybe flood the hearts of visiting Americans with that elusive sense of national security we crave.

I start to think maybe it's another kind of poem, this board of numbers. It wants to make people afraid and to console them at once;

it wants to give them the sense that they are in the middle of something larger and more powerful than they can ever understand—this traffic of drugs and bodies, this barely tethered and unquiet thing, *danger* itself, so porous and fluid. For every 3,567 immigrants caught, we imagine, there are always another ten thousand who aren't. The persistence of fear can be a useful thing. Official pronouncements are full of loud gaps and festering line breaks and margins throbbing with unspoken threats and promises.

So the conversation continues. Drug lords write messages on corpses, and these messages say *fuck you* to the border control and its 370 criminal arrests. Poets get ideas and they get visas and they get on flights to Los Angeles. They tell Americans about Mexicans in a little barrio called Comales. They get home and the cartels are exploding grenades that tell them: *Stay home and shut up.* Everyone is trying to talk loudest. Everyone is simply hungry for the chance to speak.

As we drive away from dawn, toward San Diego, Marco tells me about another piece he made just after the August massacre. It was designed to resemble his local yellow pages. It listed all the stores and services named for the Gulf: Siderúrgica del Golfo, El Restaurán del Golfo, Transportes Línea del Golfo. In the spot where El Cártel del Golfo would have fallen, the line read: *Puede Anunciarse Aquí.* Addressed to the cartel, to its rivals, to its victims: You Can Advertise Here.

MORPHOLOGY
⁑ OF THE HIT ⁑

We begin with the first function.

I. *One of the Members Absents Himself from Home.*

I didn't exactly leave home for Nicaragua. I'd been leaving home for years. Nicaragua was just the farthest I'd gone.

Near a city called Granada I taught Spanish to kids who knew their language better than I ever would. I worked in a school with two concrete classrooms sometimes invaded by goats or stray dogs. The dogs were skinny. Some of the kids were too, though they were always buying treats from an old woman who sold old bags of old potato chips and bright pink cookies from huge straw baskets. She sat in the shadows beside their rusty swings.

I liked the kids. They touched me—literally, my arms, legs, my whole body—more than anyone else I'd known. I knew their families by sight and sometimes by name. Many of their mothers sold chewing gum and cashews in the *parque central* next to the bus station. Their fathers and brothers called out *"¡Guapa chica!"* every time I passed. I should have been offended. I wasn't.

I turned twenty-four in a bar called *Café Bohemia*. I made sangria with local fruits and wrote notes from the Internet café that said: *I made sangria with local fruits!* I told everyone I was enjoying the easy commonality of being a foreigner among foreigners: *None of us are where we usually are!* I said. *We are lost together!* The keyboard was strangely arranged under my fingers. I still hadn't gotten used to it. It made me confuse certain punctuation marks. *Fruits from the market?* my notes said. *We are lost together?*

I never know how to start this story. I just don't. That's why I need functions. That's why maybe we need to go back further. Vladimir Propp was a man who lived in Russia through the Revolution and two wars. He wrote a book called *Morphology of the Folktale* that no one talks about much these days, except to disagree with it. It's basically a map for storytelling, a catalog of plot pieces arranged into thirty-one functions: commencements, betrayals, resolutions.

Propp's elaborate system of classifications—letters, numerals, headings, subheadings—pegs these plot points like taxidermy specimens: *trickery, guidance, rescue.* They mark moments where the action takes a different direction. Propp claims that you can break any story into an accumulation of these parts shuffled into constant rearrangements. Essentially, he is making a claim about disruptions. He says everything proceeds from losing our place.

III. *The Interdiction Is Violated.*

Now we're out of order and we've hardly begun. Propp maps imperfectly onto the story. I keep coming back to his functions anyway. This is the third one. This interdiction was an old one: Girls should never be alone in the dark. This is wisdom from the fairy tales.

Afterward they said I shouldn't have been walking at night. In that neighborhood. On an empty street, alone. Here's what "alone" really means: without a man.

It was mainly men, saying this last one.

Some said it kindly. Others sounded annoyed. The point is nobody had really said it before. Which means we'll have to rearrange the functions. We return to the second after the violation of the third.

II. *An Interdiction Is Addressed to the Hero.*

I hadn't been instructed not to walk alone. I'd been instructed not to be afraid. Granada was safe. Nicaragua wasn't just violence. That was an idea that belonged to Americans, the ones who didn't know any better.

This is the function that baptizes the hero. Its pair of points—the rule and its transgression—is what makes him a hero in the first place.

My prohibition was fear. I was told to keep my fear within bounds. Or at least keep it to myself. My friend Omar said: "All of you are so afraid here."

All of you: women, Americans, visitors. I was all of these, but I would learn not to be. I'd learn how to be different, try harder, walk through the streets without watching for some stranger in the shadows. I'd arrived somewhere I'd never been invited.

For starters, there was the question of history. Which wasn't my fault, exactly, but did make me involved. The history was studded with absurdities: the Contra War, the arms scandal. Reagan everything. Bush everything. Omar recited the best bits of Bush's debates with Hugo Chavez—Chavez, still something of a hero in that country—and I laughed louder than anyone. I hated Bush too. I needed them to know that.

Maybe I didn't have the right to need anything from that place. Maybe that didn't make it right that I got punched in the face. But maybe I wasn't entirely innocent, either.

So now I've given away the ending. I got punched.

I'm still looking for the proper function for this part. What is morphology anyway? I looked it up and found this: "The study of the shape or form of things."

Which is how we keep something trapped in its place: we give it a form.

Maybe VI. *The Villain Attempts to Deceive His Victim in Order to Take Possession of Him or of His Belongings.*

There was no trickery. Only a man coming at me from behind, turning me around, hitting me hard. No deception. One of the most honest gestures I'd ever seen.

Maybe V. *The Villain Receives Information about His Victim.*

Propp cites examples. The many species of reconnaissance: Spies are sent. Hiding places are found. A villainous bear uses a talking chisel to find some missing children.

On that street in Nicaragua it was simpler. A man was sitting on the curb beside a vacant *lavandería*. He saw me and he sized me up, just like that: *Gringa. Chica.* Tourist.

Guapa chica, they said—other men, on the streets. But he said nothing.

Who knows what he thought? I just know this: whatever he saw—whatever he thought he saw—it was enough.

So here it is.

Function VIII. *The Villain Causes Harm or Injury.*

I was punched. I bled all over my arms, my legs, my skirt, my shoes. I wasn't crying. I was speaking. What was I saying?

I was saying: "I'm okay I'm okay I'm okay."

I was saying: "There is so much blood."

Propp says: "This function is exceptionally important." He says: "The forms of villainy are exceedingly varied."

Here are some of them: *The villain pillages or spoils the crops, the villain causes a sudden disappearance, the villain casts a spell, the villain threatens forced matrimony, the villain makes a threat of cannibalism.*

Here are two more: *The villain seizes the daylight. The villain torments at night.*

"The city is different at night," Omar had said. "Everything is possible."

Some functions describe villains stealing body parts. You break something and you steal the way it used to look. That never comes back.

"He took your wallet?" someone asked me. "And your camera?" I nodded. I wanted to say: *he took my face.*

Here are some functions missing from my story: *The Seeker Agrees to or Decides upon Counteraction, The Hero Reacts to the Actions, The Hero and Villain Join in Direct Combat.*

These don't apply to me.

This one does: XVII. *The Hero Is Branded.*

My nose was broken. The bones of the bridge got shifted. The flesh swelled like it was trying to hide the fracture beneath. This is how speech swells around memory. How intellect swells around hurt.

XIV. *The Hero Acquires the Use of a Magical Agent.*

Meaning what? The Nicaraguan police? The liquor I drank—shots and then more of them—to make myself feel all right again, to make myself stop shaking?

After the hit, I went to a bar on Calle Calzada. I knew the guys who worked there. They saw me right off and knew what I needed. They'd been in fights. This kind of injury wasn't anything new. They gave me wet rags, ice, a beer. I kept putting all three against my face, very gently. I wasn't sure if my nose was loose enough to push out of place. I couldn't even look them in the eye. I was ashamed. I wouldn't be able to explain this properly to anyone. It had something to do with being seen. Everything was visible to them—swollen face, bloody arms, bloody legs, bloody clothes. These were the only things I was composed of, and everyone saw them—everyone understood them—as well as I could. It was a kind of nakedness, a feeling of nerve endings in the wind.

The police showed up in a pickup truck with a large cage strapped to the back. There was a man inside the cage. I was sitting on the curb with my rags and my beer. The cop was smoking a cigarette. He pointed to the man in the cage: "¿Es el hombre?"

This wasn't the man. This was just *a* man. I hadn't even given them a description.

I shook my head. The cop shrugged. He let the man go. The man seemed angry. Of course he did.

That cop was nice, but he never expected things to go any other way than the way they went. He showed me huge leather volumes of mug shots, sepia-toned portraits of local street thugs with their nicknames written in spidery cursive underneath: *el toro, el caballero, el serpiente.*

None of them were him. I said: "No, no, no."

I went to the police station the next morning. It was a ratty building with brown stains on the walls and a broken toilet you could smell from all the other rooms. Or someone could, at least. I couldn't smell anything. There were old typewriters on most of the desks and a few broken ones stacked in the corner. The station was in a part of town I'd never seen. It wasn't a part of town that tourists would have any reason to visit unless they were there to complain. I'd been living in Nicaragua for several months, and I'd never felt more like a tourist than I did right then, part of a story everyone had heard before.

The cops were eager to show off their new face-profiling software. I sat with one guy at a computer—one of the only ones, it seemed, in the whole station. He asked me questions about what the guy looked like and I answered them badly. "He had eyebrows," I may have said—did I say? I was waiting for adjectives to offer themselves up. But none came. The sketch on the computer screen looked nothing like the man.

XXIX. *The Hero Is Given a New Appearance.*

Propp gets more explicit: "A new appearance is directly effected by means of the magical actions of a helper." I got back to Los Angeles and saw a surgeon. There was something in my face that wasn't right. Anyone could see that. I wanted it fixed. I felt sick with self-preservation. The surgeon looked at my face and said: "Something happened to you."

"I know," I said. "Can you fix it?"

He said: "I can't tell from outside."

So he went in. I went under.

I still get stuck on this one, a few functions back: XIX. *The Initial Misfortune or Lack Is Liquidated.*

Propp says: "The narrative reaches its peak in this function."

What does this function feel like? I'm still waiting for it.

The surgery got rid of the break. Or else it got rid of the evidence. But I can still find the slant if I look for it, the diagonal remains of fist hitting bone.

You can find a program on the Internet called "Digital Propp." I guess you'd call it a game. You click on the site and it says: "You have reached the Proppian Fairy Tale Generator, an experiment in electronic (re)writing and an exploration of the retranslation of modernist theory within the electronic environment."

Here's what you do. You check off the functions you want and it gives you a story. I check: *absentation, interdiction, violation, villainy, branding, exposure.* I pause, go back, check off: *lack.*

I don't check: *counteraction, recognition, wedding.*

I click the little button called "generate." The site spits back a story: something about a forbidden pear, and then some fight with a bird, some victory having to do with flying. I'm seeing signs of all kinds of functions I didn't ask for: struggle, challenge, victory. There is some fighting and finally some winning: "The soil on my skin turned into sprinkles of gold dust. The people proclaimed me some kind of god."

The materials of my life, as memory recalls and deforms them, will always involve him: the stranger. Maybe our union replaces my final neglected function: XXXI. *The Hero Is Married and Ascends the Throne.* I wanted a man to fall in love with me so he could get angry about how I'd gotten hit. I wasn't supposed to want this. I wanted it anyway.

Months later I saw an ex-boyfriend in Williamsburg and he offered me a line of coke on someone's steamer trunk. I imagined my nose dissolving right off my face.

I shook my head.

He said: "Why not?"

I told him why not. He stopped smiling. He got very upset. It felt like he wanted something from me. What did he want? I didn't know what I could give him.

When I got back from Nicaragua and tried to explain what had happened to me, I felt like I was constantly shuffling together pieces of an elaborate puzzle I couldn't see the edges of: violence, randomness, impersonality and swollen face, pure cash and tourist guilt. Guilt always sounded wrong—like I was trying to apologize for what had happened, or say that my status as a tourist somehow justified it—when I wasn't trying to excuse anything, only to speak a feeling of culpability tangled with the other kinds of residue inside me: anger, fear, an obsessive tendency to check the mirror for signs that my parts were slipping out of place. I began graduate school and started writing papers about the practice of rereading. I read Propp. I looked back at my own life like text.

There is no function designated for this last part. This present tense, when the hero turns to some archaic work of early Russian

Formalism to understand how her face was hurt, how something quiet happened to the rest of her as well.

There is no function designated for how this essay might begin to fill the lack or liquidate the misfortune—replace the eyes, the heart, the daylight. Everything I find is stained by a certain residue: all that blood. My face will always remind me of a stranger. And I will never know his name.

‡ PAIN TOURS (I) ‡

La Plata Perdida

This is how you visit the silver mines of Potosí, the highest city in the world: First take an airplane to El Alto, where some people's hearts collapse under the altitude as soon as they step off the plane. El Alto is at 4,061 meters. Potosí is higher. You take a bus to Ororu, and another one from there. You might share your seat with an animal. You might see a movie starring Jean-Claude Van Damme. These are popular on overnights: Van Damme fighting terrorists, killing bad guys, speaking the mouth-awkward language of another dubbed tongue.

When you get off the bus, Potosí will look like other Bolivian towns—old women roasting ears of corn over open flames, sidewalks full of skinny dogs and broken appliances—until it looks different: the pastel walls around its central plaza, the elegant balconies, the stately courtyards. Maybe you think it's beautiful. Maybe you think it's too much, too colonial, a little gauche. Maybe later, the memory of these buildings will make you feel a bit sick in the heart.

People come to Potosí to see the famous silver mines of Cerro Rico, so you will see them too. Take a tour. Smile politely when the man behind the desk tells you that the miners will get a cut of the money. Tell him, in your beseeching Spanish, that this is very nice. Put on your gear: boots and overalls, a bandanna over your mouth. Take a van to the miners' market. Here, you will find severed goats' heads sharing tables with Che Guevara ski caps. ¡Viva la Revolución! There are shiny white skins, unfurled, that are the long stripped interiors of animals' intestines.

But you are here to buy presents for the underground men: bright sodas whose flavors are colors instead of fruits; sticks of dynamite; coca leaves in small blue bags. These are gifts for the miners but really, of course, they are gifts for the givers: you will *give something back*, as they say, and this pleases you. You will cover your subterranean tracks.

Listen carefully to your guide, Favio, an angry man your own age. He is barely twenty-five but he has three brothers in the mines and two young sons who will work here too, someday, unless he can pay their way out. Then he smiles slightly and says, *"but you did not come to hear about my life,"* and you did, of course, always greedy for other people's lives, but first you must listen to the rest because listening is a gift too, or this is what you tell yourself: the tentative idea that this knowing can make a difference.

So *¡oye!* Listen up. They call Cerro Rico the mountain that eats men because it already has, six million so far. Potosí *conquistadores* got rich on its silver and they built all kinds of pretty courtyards in town. But six million, my God. You glance sheepishly at your gifts: your lucky dynamite, your grape soda.

The mountain is full of mouths but you only visit one: a dark hole on a hillside littered with crusty old jeans, long discarded, dirty beer bottles and toilet paper, small mounds of human excrement. Here, you are told, is where the miners eat and drink and shit between back-to-back twelve-hour shifts. *Oh, yes; yes, of course.*

You find the mineshaft bearable at first, a cool dark hallway, until it absolutely isn't: two-ton trolleys barreling down thin infrastructure, steep tunnels full of foul dust, all of them snaking toward the center of an unbelievable heat. Sometimes you have to kneel. Sometimes you have to crawl. Sometimes you pass miners, cheeks bulged with mounds of half-chewed coca, and someone gives them bottles of soda while the guide asks: "How are you?"

Favio gives you the scoop on President Evo. Everybody thought he'd make it better but then he didn't. Evo calls the miners his brothers but still keeps raising their taxes. There have been strikes.

There have always been strikes. Things are "under discussion" in
La Paz. You nod. You know there must be questions worth asking but what you ask is: "How much longer until we get to level
three?" You are having a little trouble breathing. Your bandanna is
gummed with gray dust.

In level three, at the end of the ventilation tubes, you see two
men standing at the bottom of a dark hole. "Let me tell you how we
get through the day," Favio says. "We miners, we are always telling
jokes. These men were probably telling jokes just before we came."
They have been underground for five hours and they've got another
seven left. Do they want some dynamite, as a gift? They do.

On the way out, you pass the statue of a demon. He is called
Tío. The Uncle-Devil. He's got a cigarette in his mouth, a beer in
his hand, and a big wooden erection in his crotch. The miners are
mainly Catholic but down here they worship the devil. Who else
could possibly hold sway? They worship until they are thirty-five, or
maybe forty, and then they die. They die from accidents or silicosis,
a disease one calls "the uniting of dust in the lungs." They leave their
sons behind to work a mountain with a little less silver than the one
their fathers worked, and their fathers before them.

At the exit, there is sunlight and clean air. This is something. But
you catch sight of yourself in the darkened glass of your minivan—
your cheeks black, neck black, lips black—and the truth is you look
like a devil too.

Sublime, Revised

The warning, as ever, is also a promise: *This program contains subject matter and language that may be disturbing to some viewers.* It's
a promise the same way an ambulance is a promise, or a scar, or a
freeway clogged around an accident.

The show is called *Intervention,* and each episode is named for
its addict: Jimbo, Cassie, Benny, Jenna. Danielle lines up twelve pre-
scription bottles on the coffee table while her eight-year-old says,

"I know real mommy is just waiting to come out." Sonia and Julia are anorexic twins who follow each other around the house so that one won't burn more calories than the other. Everyone has a wound: Gloria drinks because of her breast cancer. Danielle takes her mother's Percocet because her father is a drunk. Marci drinks because she lost custody of her kids because she drinks.

Andrea is twenty-nine. She hasn't lived with her husband and children for nine months. She spends her days drinking rum carefully rationed by her mother. She takes a drink and tells her mother, "This one is because you never got me counseling." She keeps a bottle of Captain Morgan in one hand and a liter of Pepsi in the other. She has bruises all over her body from where she's tripped over chairs, fallen into door frames, landed on the floor. Excessive bruising can be a sign of compromised liver function, the show tells us. We are given scientists' eyes. We can see the purpling damage for ourselves.

The camera work is an experiment in turning monotony into something interesting. The fatigue and stamina of addiction are kept electric by compression: time-lapse shots of a bottle's sinking line of whiskey; a cancerous pile of empties in the corner; a timeline of photos that ticks off stations of the cross, sinner to martyr to corpse: smiling baby gives way to pockmarked meth ghoul gives way to sullen mug shot.

Sober Andrea talks about her responsibilities. Drunk Andrea talks about her afflictions. She toasts the twin nodes of trauma that constitute her life: an absent alcoholic father and a rape at fourteen. When she is drunk, she doesn't believe she can do anything but hurt.

The structure of the show implicitly endorses her narrative of victimhood. It needs a story to tell, after all, and she's fashioned one—a story patterned by the saving, satisfying grace of cause-and-effect: get raped, get silenced, get abandoned, get drunk. The television program needs a genealogy for her dysfunction. Getting drunk is more interesting when it can be read as a ledger of traumas rather than their source. Recovering alcoholics sometimes talk about feeling like they never got the Life Instruction Manual everyone else got. Here's a substitute set of imperatives: lose a job, get drunk; lose a child, get drunker. Lose everything. Andrea has. So get sober. Maybe she will.

The father of her children, Jason, barely greets her when she comes to visit the kids each month. She still calls him the love of her life. He says, "What's up?" and keeps cooking lunch. He declines to be interviewed by the program. He doesn't participate in the intervention. He's given up. He's not crying on the other side of the bathroom door, or yanking the bottle from her hands. He's just gone.

We're not gone, though, we viewers. We stay with Andrea after she tells her children good-bye. We see her get drunk, again. We see why it might have been hard for Jason to stay.

The shows takes care to emphasize, over and over again, that the participants have agreed to be on a reality TV show about addiction but don't know they will face an intervention. Given that the biggest reality TV show about addiction in America today is *Intervention*, this is a bit difficult to believe. But the point is, people want to believe it. They want to know something the addict doesn't. They want the intervention to be climactic, surprising, and powerful. They want to be in on it. *Don't throw your life away, Andrea,* they'd say, if they were in the room. *I think you can make it.*

In his theory of the sublime, eighteenth-century philosopher Edmund Burke proposes the notion of "negative pain": the idea that a feeling of fear—paired with a sense of safety, and the ability to look away—can produce a feeling of delight. One woman can sit on her couch with a glass of Chardonnay and watch another woman drink away her life. The TV is a portal that brings the horror close, and a screen that keeps it at bay—revising Burke's sublime into a sublime voyeurism, no longer awe at the terrors of nature but fascination at the depths of human frailty.

The professionals who moderate the show's interventions are called "Interventionists," a title that seems better suited to a blockbuster film about the Apocalypse. I imagine a slick troop of heroes, clad in black, giving an ultimatum to the world about its addiction to

capitalism or oil. These Interventionists are mild-mannered grand-
parents dressed in business casual. They almost always stress the
singularity of the intervention—"You will never get another chance
like this," they say. They mean what they hope: this moment will
divide the addict's life into a cleanly spliced Before and After.

It's true, of course: the addict will probably never get another
intervention like this—which is to say, on reality TV—but this is
precisely the difference between the addict and his audience. For
the regular viewer, the once-in-a-lifetime intervention happens every
Monday night at nine. The unrepeatable is repeated. Every week is
a relapse, the viewer thrown back into addiction after last week's
vow to stay clean. Epiphany is succeeded by another intoxication. A
grown woman throws up on her mother's couch once more. A needle
jams into the same junked vein. Disturbance is promised, recorded,
dissolved—then resurrected, so it can be healed again.

Indigenous to the Hood

Start the Gang Tour at a Silverlake building called the Dream
Center, where grown adults cluster around the bus like kids on a
field trip. Pay sixty-five dollars and take a complimentary bottled
water. Notice the church group from Missouri, twenty-strong and
blond, and eye their grocery bag full of snacks: Teddy Grahams,
Pringles, Cheetos. Notice the surprising number of Australians.
They pace restlessly. One of them is named Tiny, but he isn't. He appears to be here with his son, a teenager in baggy shorts and braces.

Alfred is the tour's founder and guide. He's a marine turned
gangbanger turned entrepreneur. He's cracking Inner City Jokes.
His phrase. Like: "We don't need the windows open cuz we don't
do drive-bys." Also, we can't have them open because the bus is
air-conditioned. Alfred has hired three other guys to help lead the
tour—ex-gang members who had trouble finding other jobs with
felonies on their records. They've turned their experiences into stories for travelers. They are curators and exhibits at once. When
they're not giving tours, they're doing conflict mediation in the

communities these tours put on display. Your sixty-five dollars will fund this work.

Your friend the screenwriter arrives bearing a half-drunk chai that disappointed him. He compliments your tactful yellow dress, neither Crips blue nor Bloods red, and you remember elementary school field trips downtown. You and your fellow Westsiders were given careful instructions about gang hues. Your subconscious still follows them. The Missouri group leader is a buzz-cut guy whom Alfred affectionately calls Pastor. "Where's Pastor?" he says, when he's talking about something Pastor might be interested in.

On board the bus, the jokes continue—"In the event of an emergency, you'll find bulletproof vests under your seats"—but the scenery changes. Silverlake bungalows give way to the warehouses of downtown and the signage of a hybrid city—papuserías and pho shops, Spanglish enticements: *Thrift Store y Café.* 1-800-72-DADDY promises dads it can get them custody or at least visitation rights.

Each guide stands at the front of the bus to tell his story. One guy, let's call him Capricorn, points out the projects where his first girlfriend still lives. "Still won't take my calls," he says. Another guy lays down statistics: every felony, every sentence, every prison, how much coke he got busted for each time. One guy describes a brutal turf war on the first day of junior high, when the kids from three different elementary schools—each one loyal to a different gang— were all jammed together for the first time. They started clapping at each other until the police came. You think clapping is a kind of hand signal. You learn it's not. You learn boys get their first guns when they're eleven or twelve.

You hear notes of something like nostalgia when these guys talk about their former lives—the weapons and arrests, the monstrous tallies of their cash flows. Pride comes before the fall and also after it. But the nostalgia is tangled up with a deep and genuine lamenting of the terms of this territory—how harshly it circumscribes the path, how inevitably it punishes alternatives. Things are different now, though. These men got out of prison and wanted another

way. When Alfred says, "I'm a spiritual man," you see him looking around to see if Pastor's listening. His reform is operative on all
fronts. He'll tell you about his struggle for a bigger vocabulary: "I
learned 'gentrification' in solitary"; "I practice pronouncing 'recidi-
vism' in the shower." He calls Capricorn's life story "an indigenous
tale from the hood."

Scholar Graham Huggan defines "exoticism" as an experience
that "posits the lure of difference while protecting its practitioners
from close involvement." You're in the hood but you aren't—it rolls
by your windows, a perfect panorama of itself. *We don't do drive-bys.*
You just drive by.

You pass the old LA County jail, which is surprisingly beautiful. It's got a handsome stone facade and stately columns. The
new LA County jail—called the Twin Towers—isn't beautiful at
all; it's a stucco panopticon the color of sick flesh. Alfred gets on
the mic to talk about his time in there: ten guys in a cell designed
for six, extra men moved to closets and kitchens whenever inspection teams rolled through. He talks about the rats. He calls them
Freeway Freddies. It was an ecosystem in there, and out here too:
you see an entire neighborhood selling bail bonds. You see Abba
Bail Bonds and Jimmie Dright Jr. Bail Bonds and Big Dog a.k.a. *I'm
still tough* Bail Bonds, and Aladdin a.k.a. *I need my fucking third wish*
Bail Bonds. Bail bond shops remind you that every guy serving time
has a mother and every mother probably has a story of that time she
went to the bail bond strip mall and had no idea which bail bond
shop to choose.

From downtown, you head to South Central and finally to Watts.
The towers are eerie and wondrous, like something a witch made,
pointing ragged into a blue sky. Capricorn tells you he's climbed
them. Most kids in Watts have climbed them. A lot of guys get them
tattooed on their backs or biceps—the distinctive profile of their
bony cones. One of the Missouri girls asks, "What're they made of?"
and Capricorn says, "What does it look like they're made of?"

You like this kind of tour, where there is such a thing as a stupid question, though this—to you—doesn't seem like one. What

are they made of? Capricorn finally mutters, "Shells and shit." He's right, you find out later. They're made of shells, steel, mortar, glass, and pottery. An immigrant named Simon Rodia made Italian folk art the template for generations of gang tats.

Capricorn tells you he chose his name before he knew his zodiac sign. It happened to work out. He gets a call from a guy named Puppet but doesn't take it. He says, "I can't deal with that right now." He tells you he still believes his phone is tapped—by whom, he doesn't say—so he changes phones nearly every week, gives the old ones to his nieces and nephews. Your screenwriter friend says, "So now your nieces' and nephews' phones are tapped?" Capricorn doesn't laugh. Your friend tells him you grew up here, in Santa Monica, and you feel ashamed because you know Santa Monica isn't here at all.

The *here* of Watts is pastel houses with window gratings in curly patterns. *Here* is yard sales with bins full of stuffed animals and used water guns. Here is Crips turf. "Being a spectator of calamities taking place in another country," writes Susan Sontag, "is a quintessential modern experience." Part of what feels strange about this tour is that you're assuming the posture of a tourist—*How many people have died here? How do the boys come of age?*—but you are only eighteen miles from where you grew up.

Alfred says more people have died in LA gang conflicts than the Troubles in Ireland. You'd never thought of it like that, which is his point: no one thinks of it like that. These blocks look so ordinary. South Central Avenue itself is just a gritty bracelet of strip malls and auto body shops; Watts is parched lawns that once burned. The here of Watts was on fire in 1965. Black boys who hadn't gotten into the Boy Scouts were sick of it. They made their own clubs. Thirty-five thousand people rose up. People got sick of it again in 1992, when Rodney King was beaten and thousands of people, the children of the Watts riots, said *enough*. Reginald Denny with a brick to the head said *enough*.

You try to remember what you thought about Rodney King when you were young, but you can't. Is that possible? You can't. You were nine years old. You can remember, faintly, that some part of you got stubborn about the police—*but they only would've hit him if he did something wrong.* You still wanted to believe in uniforms and a system of order that had always served you well. You remember OJ Simpson better than King. OJ Simpson's wife was killed in Brentwood, where you went to school.

Rodney King was swarmed and then he was beaten. He suffered fifty-six baton blows. Two officers broke his face with their feet. Where were you back then? You were a kid. You were on the coast. Other kids had to be kids farther east, where people got angry at the corner of Florence and Normandie and stayed angry at the corner of Florence and Normandie, stayed angry at Koon and Powell and the paleness of Ventura County, and for days the fires wouldn't stop.

Your refrigerated bus crosses the concrete spine of the LA River, icon and encapsulation of the city's wasteland shame. The gray banks are covered with patches of lighter gray where paint has been layered over graffiti. Alfred points out a long stretch of painted riverbank—three stories high, and three-quarters of a mile long— where the world's biggest tag used to be. It read MTA: Metro Transit Assassins. It was visible from Google Space. Now the grayness is like a sprawling tombstone—another scar in a battle between two different structures of authority, two civic institutions trying to claim the same space.

Alfred delivers a lesson on graffiti taxonomy: the difference between tag and flare and roller, between a masterpiece and a throwup. A masterpiece has more than three colors. A throw-up usually means bubble letters but sounds more like some boy vomited the colors from his mouth. On a downtown wall, you see a painted face vomiting rainbows. Across the street, you see what looks like a polar bear illuminated by sunset. "Look at that throw-up," you tell your screenwriter friend. "Masterpiece," he corrects, pointing out five colors. You realize that three-story MTA would've been a masterpiece too. You learn that every graffiti act in the state of California is a felony. You learn that painted hot-chick skulls are called Sugar Skulls. You learn that three dots tattooed under the eye means *la vida loca,* as in: *I plan to keep living the.* You think those dots look like tears suspended against gravity. You don't know whether they signal commitment or renunciation or something in between. Tiny's teenage son asks Alfred, eager: "Were you much of a tagger?" He asks Capricorn if his family still lives in Watts, and—if so—if we'll get to see them on the tour.

The outing ends under a sultry Sugar Skull. You all pose for "gang shots" in front of a huge mural that says *Big Los Angeles* in bright blue bubble letters. Or maybe you don't pose, because you feel uncomfortable. But the Aussie guys are psyched for it, flashing their hand signs and sporting tough-guy pouts. One girl from Missouri gets some backseat posing advice from her friends—"Look tough!"—but fucks it up because she can't stop grinning. Pastor poses with the bus driver, who's taken off his shirt to show an inked-up chest that has one rose for every year spent in prison. There's not much bare skin left.

This photo shoot feels like an odd capstone. You've come to understand gang violence as symptomatic of an abiding civil conflict whose proportions we can only begin to fathom; now you watch church kids fumble their fingers toward *Eastside,* toward *Killaz.* Maybe Pastor will change his Facebook profile to a shot of himself and Capricorn gripping palm-to-palm. "Photographs objectify," Sontag writes, "they turn an event or person into something that can be possessed." Now Pastor owns a small corner of the hood—or perhaps, more to the point, he owns a moment of his own experience. He can pack up his own heightened awareness like a souvenir. His opened eyes are take-home talismans. You want the tour to give you back another version of yourself, you and everyone: a more enlightened human.

You imagine the sermon in Branson the next Sunday, Capricorn and Alfred like ghosts of glorious reform behind the pulpit. Maybe Pastor will say, *These men turned a 180 you wouldn't believe.* Maybe his congregation will break the silence with their clapping.

You'd clap for that sermon, actually. These men were raised into violence—raised *by* it, like a parent—and now they live another way. Is it possible to say—in the most full-hearted and deeply earnest sense, uncluttered by disclaimers—that this tour is impossible to look away from and important to remember?

You feel uncomfortable. Your discomfort is the point. Friction rises from an asymmetry this tour makes plain: the material of your diverting morning is the material of other people's lives, and their deaths. The unease of the tour is not the discomfort of being problematically present—South Central mediated by air-conditioning vents—so much as the discomfort of an abiding absence—a pattern of always being elsewhere, far away, out of ear- and eye- and gunshot, humming beach to bistro along the Pacific Coast Highway.

What good is this tour except that it offers an afterward? You're just a tourist inside someone else's suffering until you can't get it out of your head; until you take it home with you—across a freeway, or a country, or an ocean. No bail to post: everything lingers. Puppet lingers. Those clapping seventh graders linger. Your own embarrassment lingers. Maybe moral outrage is just the culmination of an insoluble lingering. So prepare yourself to live in it for a while. Hydrate for the ride. The great shame of your privilege is a hot blush the whole time. The truth of this place is infinite and irreducible, and self-reflexive anguish might feel like the only thing you can offer in return. It might be hard to hear anything above the clattering machinery of your guilt. Try to listen anyway.

THE IMMORTAL
⁑ HORIZON ⁑

On the western edge of Frozen Head State Park, just before dawn, a man in a rust-brown trench coat blows a giant conch shell. Runners stir in their tents. They fill their water pouches. They tape their blisters. They eat thousand-calorie breakfasts: Pop-Tarts and candy bars and geriatric energy drinks. Some of them pray. Others ready their fanny packs. The man in the trench coat sits in an ergonomic lawn chair beside a famous yellow gate, holding a single cigarette. He calls the two-minute warning.

The runners gather in front of him, stretching. They are about to travel a hundred miles through the wilderness—if they are strong and lucky enough to make it that far, which they probably aren't. They wait anxiously. We, the watchers, wait anxiously. Pale light bleeds faintly across the sky. Next to me, a skinny girl holds a skinny dog. She has come all the way from Iowa to watch her father disappear into this gray dawn.

All eyes are on the man in the trench coat. At precisely 7:12, he rises from his lawn chair and lights his cigarette. Once the tip glows red, the race known as the Barkley Marathons has begun.

The first race was a prison break. On June 11, 1977, James Earl Ray, the man who shot Martin Luther King Jr., escaped from Brushy Mountain State Penitentiary and fled across the briar-bearded hills of northern Tennessee. Fifty-one-and-a-half hours later he was found. He'd gone about two kilometers. Some might hear this and wonder how he managed to squander his escape. One man heard this and thought: *I need to see that terrain!*

Twenty years later, that man, the man in the trench coat—Gary

Cantrell by birth, self-dubbed Lazarus Lake—has turned this terrain into the stage for a legendary ritual: the Barkley Marathons, held yearly (traditionally on either Lazarus Friday or April Fool's Day) outside Wartburg, Tennessee. Lake (known as Laz) calls it "The Race That Eats Its Young." The runners' bibs say something different each year: *Suffering without a point; Not all pain is gain.* Only eight men have ever finished. The event is considered extreme even by those who specialize in extremity.

What makes it so bad? No trail, for one. A cumulative elevation gain that's nearly twice the height of Everest. Native flora called saw briars that can turn a man's legs to raw meat in meters. The tough hills have names like Rat Jaw, Little Hell, Big Hell, Testicle Spectacle—this last so-called because it inspires most runners to make the sign of the cross (crotch to eyeglasses, then shoulder to shoulder)—not to mention Stallion Mountain, Bird Mountain, Coffin Springs, Zipline, and an uphill stretch, new this year, known simply as "The Bad Thing."

The race consists of five loops on a course that's been officially listed at twenty miles but is probably more like twenty-six. The moral of this slanted truth is that standard metrics are irrelevant. The moral of a lot of Barkley's slanted truths is that standard metrics are irrelevant. The laws of physics and human tolerance have been replaced by Laz's personal whims. Even if the race were really "only" a hundred miles, these would still be "Barkley miles." Guys who could typically finish a hundred miles in twenty hours might not finish a single loop here. If you finish three, you've completed what's known as the Fun Run. If you happen *not* to finish—and, let's face it, you probably won't—Laz will play bugle Taps to commemorate your quitting. The whole camp, shifting and dirty and tired, will listen, except for those who are asleep or too weak to notice, who won't.

It's no easy feat to get here. There are no published entry requirements or procedures. It helps to know someone. Admissions are decided by Laz's personal discretion, and his application isn't exactly standard, with questions like "What is your favorite parasite?" and a required essay with the subject: "Why I Should Be Allowed to Run the Barkley." Only thirty-five entrants are admitted. This year, one of them is my brother.

Julian is a "virgin," one of fifteen newbies who will do their damnedest to finish a loop. He has managed to escape the designation of "human sacrifice," officially applied to the virgin each year (usually the least experienced ultrarunner) whom Laz has deemed most likely to fail in a spectacular fashion—to get lost for so long, perhaps, that he manages to beat Dan Baglione's course record for slowest pace: at the age of seventy-five, in 2006, he managed two miles in thirty-two hours. Something to do with an unscrewed flashlight cap, an unexpected creek.

It's probably a misnomer to talk about getting lost at Barkley. It might be closer to the truth to say you *begin* lost, remain lost through several nights in the woods, and must constantly use your compass, map, instructions, fellow runners, and remaining shards of sanity to perpetually un-lose yourself again. First-timers usually try to stay with veterans who know the course, but are often scraped. "Virgin scraping" means ditching the new guy. A virgin bends down to tie his shoelaces, perhaps, and glances up to find his veteran Virgil gone.

The day before the race, runners start arriving at camp like rainbowed seals, sleekly gliding through the air in parti-colored body suits. They come in pickup trucks and rental cars, rusty vans and camper trailers. Their license plates say 100 Runnr, Ult Man, Crzy Run. They bring camouflage tents and orange hunting vests and skeptical girlfriends and acclimated wives and tiny travel towels and tiny dogs. Laz himself brings a little dog (named "Little Dog") with a black spot like a pirate's patch over one eye. Little Dog almost loses her name this year, after encountering and trying to eat an even smaller dog, the skinny one from Iowa, who turns out to be two dogs rather than just one.

It's a male scene. There are a few female regulars, I learn, but they rarely manage more than a loop. Most of the women in sight, like me, are part of someone's support crew. I help sort Julian's supplies in the back of the car.

He needs a compass. He needs pain pills and No-Doze pills and electrolyte pills and ginger chews for when he gets sleepy and a "kit" for popping blisters that basically consists of a needle and Band-Aids. He needs tape for when his toenails start falling off. He needs batteries. We pay special attention to the batteries. Running out of batteries is *the must-avoid-at-all-costs-worst-possible-thing-that-could-happen*. But it has happened. It happened to Rich Limacher, whose night spent under a huge Buckeye tree earned it the name "Limacher's Hilton." Our coup de grâce is a pair of duct-tape pants that we've fashioned in the manner of cowboy chaps. They will fend off saw briars, is the idea, and earn Julian the envy of the other runners.

Traditionally, the epicenter of camp is a chicken fire kindled on the afternoon before the race begins. This year's fire is blazing by 4:00 p.m. It's manned by someone named Doc Joe. Julian tells me he's been waitlisted for several years and (he speculates) has offered himself as a helper in order to secure a spot for 2011. We arrive just as he's spearing the first thighs from the grill. He's got a two-foot can of beans in the fire pit, already bubbling, but the stars of this show, clearly, are the birds, skin blackened and smothered in red sauce. As legend has it, the chicken here is served partway thawed, with only skins and "a bit more" cooked.

I ask Doc Joe how he plans to find the sweet spot between cooked and frozen. He looks at me like I'm stupid. That frozen chicken thing is just a rumor, he says. This will not be the last time, I suspect, that I catch Barkley at the game of crafting its own mythology.

At this particular potluck, small talk rarely stays banal for long. I fall into conversation with John Price, a bearded veteran who tells me he's sitting out the race this year, waitlisted, but has driven hundreds of miles just to be "a part of the action." Our conversation starts predictably. He asks where I'm from. I say Los Angeles. He says he loves Venice Beach. I say I love Venice Beach, too. Then he says: "Next fall I'm running from Venice Beach to Virginia Beach to celebrate my retirement."

I've learned not to pause at this kind of declaration. I've learned to proceed to practical questions. I ask: "Where will you sleep?"

"Mainly camping," he says. "A few motels."

"You'll carry the tent in a backpack?"

"God no," he laughs. "I'll be pulling a small cart harnessed to my waist."

I find myself at the picnic table, which has become a veritable bulimic's buffet, spread with store-bought cakes and sprinkle cookies and brownies. It's designed to feed men who will do little for the next few days besides burn an incredible number of calories.

The tall man next to me is tearing into a massive chicken thigh. His third, I've noticed. Its steam rises softly into the twilight.

"So that whole frozen thing?" I ask him. "It's really just a myth?"

"It *was* one year," he says. "It was honest-to-God frozen." He pauses. "Man! That year was a great race."

This guy introduces himself as Carl—broad and good looking, he's a bit less sinewy than many of his fellow runners. He tells me he runs a machine shop down in Atlanta. As best I can gather, this means he uses his machines to build *other* machines, or else he uses his machines to build things that aren't machines—like bicycle parts or flyswatters. He works by commission. "The people who ask for crazy inventions," he sighs, "are never the ones who can afford them."

Carl tells me that he's got an ax to grind this time around. He's got a strong history at Barkley—one of the few runners who has finished a Fun Run under official time—but his performance last year was dismal. "I barely left camp," he says. Translated, this means he ran only thirty-five miles. But it was genuinely disappointing: he didn't even finish a second loop. He tells me he was dead-tired and heartbroken. He'd just gone through a nasty breakup.

But now he's back. He looks pumped. I ask him who he thinks the major contenders are to complete a hundred.

"Well," he says, "there's always Blake and AT."

He means two of the "alumni" (former finishers) who are running this year: Blake Wood, class of 2001, and Andrew Thompson,
class of 2009. Finishing the hundred twice would make history.
Two years in a row is the stuff of fantasy.

Blake is a nuclear engineer at Los Alamos with a doctorate from
Berkeley and an incredible Barkley record: six for six Fun Run com-
pletions; one finish; another near-finish that was blocked only by a
flooded creek. In person, he's just a friendly middle-aged dad with a
salt-and-pepper mustache, eager to talk about his daughter's bid to
qualify for the Olympic Marathon Trials, and about the new pair
of checkered clown pants he'll wear this year to boost his spirits on
the trail.

AT is Andrew Thompson, a youngish guy from New Hampshire
famous for a near-finish in 2004, when he was strong heading into
his fifth loop but literally lost his mind when he was out there—
battered from fifty hours of sleep deprivation and physical strain.
He completely forgot about the race. He spent an hour squishing
mud in his shoes. He came back every year until he finally finished
the thing in 2009.

There's Jonathan Basham, AT's best support crew for years, at
Barkley for his own race this time around. He's a strong runner,
though I mainly hear him mentioned in the context of his relationship to AT, who calls him "Jonboy."

Though Carl doesn't say it, I learn from others that he's a strong
contender too. He's one of the toughest runners in the pack, a DNF
(Did Not Finish) veteran hungry for a win.

There are some strong virgins in the pack, including Charlie
Engle, already an accomplished ultrarunner (he's "done" the Sahara—
which, in this world, means running across it on foot). Like many
ultrarunners, he's also a former addict. He's been sober for nearly
twenty years, and his recovery has been described as the switch from
one addiction to another—drugs for adrenaline, trading that extreme
for this one.

If there's such a thing as the opposite of a virgin, it's probably

John DeWitt. He's an old man in a black ski cap, seventy-three and wrinkled, with a gruff voice that sounds like it should belong to a smoker or a cartoon grizzly bear. He tells me that his nine-year-old grandson recently beat him in a 5K. Later, I will hear him described as an animal. He's been running the race for twenty years—never managing a finish, or even a Fun Run.

I watch Laz from across the campfire. He's darkly regal in his trench coat, warming his hands over the flames. I want to meet him, but haven't yet summoned the courage to introduce myself. When I look at him I can't help thinking of *Heart of Darkness*. Like Kurtz, Laz is bald and charismatic, leader of a minor empire, trafficker in human pain. He's like a cross between the Colonel and my grandpa. There's certainly an Inner-Station splendor to his orchestration of this whole hormone extravaganza, testosterone spread like fertilizer across miles of barren and brambled wilderness.

He speaks to "his runners" with comfort and fondness, as if they are a batch of wayward sons turned feral each year at the flick of his lighter. Most have been running "for him" (their phrase) for years. All of them bring offerings. Everyone pays a $1.60 entry fee. Alumni bring Laz a pack of his favorite cigarettes (Camel filters), veterans bring a new pair of socks, and virgins are responsible for a license plate. These license plates hang like laundry at the edge of camp, a wall of clattering metal flaps. Julian has brought one from Liberia, where—in his non-superhero incarnation as a development economist—he is working on a microfinance project. I ask him how one manages to procure a spare license plate in Liberia. He tells me he asked a guy on the street and the guy said *ten dollars* and Julian gave him five and then it appeared. Laz immediately strings it in a place of honor, right in the center, and I can tell Julian is pleased.

All through the potluck, runners pore over their instructions, five single-spaced pages that tell them "exactly where to go"—though every single runner, even those who've run the course for years, will probably get lost at least once, many of them for hours at a time. It's hard for me to understand this—*can't you just do what they say?*—until

I look at the instructions themselves. They range from surprising ("the coal pond beavers have been very active this year, be careful not to fall on one of the sharpened stumps they have left") to self-evident ("all you have to do is keep choosing the steepest path up the mountain"). But the instructions tend to cite landmarks like "the ridge" or "the rock" that seem less than useful, considering. And then there's the issue of the night.

The official Barkley requirements read like a treasure hunt: there are ten books placed at various points along the course, and runners are responsible for ripping out the pages that match their race number. Laz is playful in his book choices: *The Most Dangerous Game, Death by Misadventure, A Time to Die*—even *Heart of Darkness*, a choice that vindicates all my associative impulses.

The big talk this year is about Laz's latest addition to the course: a quarter-mile cement tunnel that runs directly under the grounds of the old penitentiary. There's a fifteen-foot drop to get in, a narrow concrete shaft to climb out, and "plenty of" standing water once you're inside. There are also, rumor has it, rats the size of possums and—when it gets warmer—snakes the size of arms. Whose arms? I wonder. Most of the guys here are pretty wiry.

The seventh course book has been hung between two poles next to the old penitentiary walls. "This is almost exactly the same place James Earl Ray went over," the instructions say. And then they say: "Thanks a lot, James."

Thanks a lot, James—for getting all this business started.

Laz has given himself the freedom to start the race whenever he wants. He announces the date but offers only two guarantees: that it will begin "sometime" between midnight and noon (*thanks a lot, Laz*), and that he will blow the conch shell an hour beforehand in warning. In general, Laz likes to start before dawn.

At the start gate, Julian is wearing a light silver jacket, a pale gray skullcap, and his homemade duct-tape chaps. He looks like a robot. He disappears uphill in a flurry of camera flashes.

Immediately after the runners take off, Doc Joe and I start grill-ing waffles. Laz strolls over with his glowing cigarette, its gray cap of untapped ash quaking between his thick fingers. I introduce myself. He introduces himself. He asks us if we think anyone has noticed that he's not actually smoking. "I can't this year," he explains, "because of my leg." He has just had surgery on an artery and his circulation isn't good. Despite this he will set up a lawn chair by the finish line, just like every year, and stay awake until every competitor has either dropped or finished. Dropping, unless you drop at the single point accessible by trail, involves a five- to six-hour commute back into camp—longer at night, especially if you get lost. Which effectively means that the act of ceasing to compete in the Barkley race is harder than running most marathons.

I tell him the cigarette looks great as an accessory. Doc Joe tells him that he's safe up to a couple of packs. Doc Joe, by the way, is really a doctor.

"Well then," Laz smiles. "Guess I'll smoke the last quarter of this one." He finishes the cigarette and then tosses it into our cooking fire, where it smokes right into our breakfast. I am aware that Laz has already been turned into a myth, and that I will probably become another one of his mythmakers. Various tropes of masculinity are at play in Laz's persona—bad-ass, teenager, father, demon, warden—and this Rubik's cube of grit and edges seems to be what Barkley's all about.

I realize Laz and I will have many hours to spend in each other's company. The runners are out on their loops anywhere from eight to thirty-two hours. Between loops, if they're continuing, they stop at camp for a few moments of food and rest. This is both succor and sadism; the oasis offers respite and temptation at once. It's the Lotus Eater's dilemma: hard to leave a good thing behind.

I use these hours without the runners to ask Laz everything I can about the race. I start with the start: how does he choose the time? He laughs uneasily. I backtrack, apologizing: would it ruin the mystery to tell me?

"One time I started at three," he says, as if in answer. "That was fun."

"Last year you started at noon, right? I heard the runners got a little restless."

"Sure did." He shakes his head, smiling at the memory. "Folks were just standing around getting antsy."

"Was it fun watching them agonize?" I ask.

"Little bit frightening, actually," he says. "Like watching a mob turn ugly."

As we speak, he mentions sections of the course—Dave's Danger Climb, Raw Dog Falls, Pussy Ridge—as if I'd know them by heart. I ask whether Rat Jaw is called that because the briars are like a bunch of little rodent teeth. He says no, it has to do with the topographic profile on a map: it reminded him of—well, of a rat jaw. I think to myself: *a lot of things might remind you of a rat jaw.* The briar scratches are known as rat bites. Laz once claimed that the briars wouldn't give you scratches any worse than the ones you'd get from baptizing a cat.

I ask about Meth Lab Hill, wondering what its topographic profile could possibly resemble.

"That's easy," he says. "First time we ran it we saw a meth lab."

"Still operating?"

"Yep," he laughs. "Those suckers thought they'd never get found. Bet they were thinking: who the *fuck* would possibly come over this hill?"

I begin to see why Laz has been so vocal about his new sections: the difficulty of The Bad Thing, the novelty of the prison tunnel. They mark his power over the terrain.

Laz has endured quite a bit of friction with park officials over the years. The race was nearly shut down for good by a man named Jim Fyke, who was upset about erosion and endangered plants. Laz simply rerouted the course around protected areas and called the detour "Fyke's Folly."

I can sense Laz's nostalgia for wilder days—when Frozen Head was still dense with the ghosts of fled felons and outlaws, thick with undiscovered junkies and their squirreled-away cold medicine.

THE EMPATHY EXAMS

Times are different now, tamer. Just last year the Rangers cut the briars on Rat Jaw a week before the race. Laz was pissed. This year, he made them promise to wait until April.

His greatest desire seems to be to devise an unrunnable race, to sustain the immortal horizon of an unbeatable challenge with contours fresh and unknowable. After the first year, when no one even came close to finishing, Laz wrote an article headlined: "The 'Trail' Wins the Barkley Marathons." It's not hard to imagine how Laz, reclining on his lawn chair, might consider the course itself his avatar: his race is a competitor strong enough to triumph, even when he can barely stand.

He used to run this race, in days of better health, but never managed to finish it. Instead, he's managed to garner respect as a man of principle—a man so committed to the notion of pain that he's willing to rally men in its pursuit.

There are only two public trails that intersect the course: Lookout Tower, at the end of South Mac Trail, and Chimney Top. Laz discourages meeting runners while they're running. "Even just the sight of other human beings is a kind of aid," he explains. "We want them to feel the full weight of their aloneness."

That said, a woman named Cathie—who looks like an ordinary housewife but is also one of a handful of veteran female "loopers"—recommends Chimney Top for a hike.

"I broke my arm there in January," she says, "but it's pretty."

"Sounds fun," I say.

"Was it that old log over the stream?" Laz asks wistfully, as if remembering an old friend.

She shakes her head.

He asks: "Was Raw Dog with you when you did it?"

"Yep."

"Was he laughing?"

A man who appears to be her husband, presumably "Raw Dog," pipes in: "Her arm was in an S-shape, Laz. I wasn't laughing."

Laz considers this for a moment. Then he asks her: "Did it hurt?"

"Think I blocked it out," she laughs. "But I heard I was cussing the whole way down the mountain."

I watch Laz shift modes fluidly between calloused *maestro* and den father. "After nightfall," he assures Doc Joe, "there *will* be carnage," but then he bends down to pet his pirate dog. "You hungry, Little?" he asks. "You might have got a lot of love today, but you still need to eat." Whenever I see him around camp, he says: "You think Julian is having fun out there?" and I finally say: "I fucking hope not!" and he smiles: *This girl gets it.*

But I can't help thinking his question dissolves precisely the kind of loneliness he seems so interested in producing, and his runners so interested in courting. The idea that when you are alone out there, someone back at camp is *thinking of you alone out there,* is— of course—just another kind of connection. Which is part of the point of this, right? That the hardship facilitates a shared solitude, an utter isolation that has been experienced before, by others, and will be experienced again, that these others are present in spirit even if the wilds have tamed or aged or brutalized or otherwise removed their bodies.

When Julian comes in from his first loop, it's almost dark. He's been out for twelve hours. I feel like I'm sharing this moment of triumph with Laz, in some sense, though I also know he's promiscuous in this sort of sharing. There's a place in his heart for everyone who runs his gauntlet, and everyone silly enough to spend days in the woods just to watch someone touch a yellow gate.

Julian is in good spirits. He turns over his pages to be counted. He's got ten 61s, including one from *The Power of Positive Thinking,* which came early in the course, and one from an account of teenage alcoholism called *The Late Great Me,* which came near the end. I notice the duct tape has been ripped from his pants. "You took it off?" I ask.

"Nope," he says. "Course took it off."

In camp he eats hummus sandwiches and Girl Scout cookies,

barely manages to gulp down a Butter Pecan Ensure. He is debating another loop. "I'm sure I won't finish," he says. "I'll probably just go out for hours and then drop and have to find my way back in the dark."

Julian pauses. I take one of his cookies.

He says: "I guess I'll do it."

He takes the last cookie before I can grab it. He takes another bib number, for his second round of pages, and Laz and I send him into the woods. His rain jacket glows silver in the darkness: brother robot, off for another spin.

Julian has completed five hundred-mile races so far, as well as countless "short" ones, and I once asked him why he does it. He explained it like this: he wants to achieve a completely insular system of accountability, one that doesn't depend on external feedback. He wants to run a hundred miles when no one knows he's running, so that the desire to impress people, or the shame of quitting, won't constitute his sources of motivation. Perhaps this kind of thinking is what got him his PhD at the age of twenty-five. It's hard to say. Barkley doesn't offer a pure form of this isolated drive, but it comes pretty close: when it's midnight and it's raining and you're on the steepest hill you've ever climbed and you're bleeding from briars and you're alone and you've been alone for hours, it's only *you* around to witness yourself quit or continue.

At four in the morning, the fire is bustling. A few frontrunners are in camp preparing to head onto their third loops, gulping coffee or taking fifteen-minute naps in their tents. It's as if the thought of the "full weight of loneliness" has inspired an urge toward companionship back here, the same way Julian's hunger—when he stops for aid—makes me feel hungry, though I have done little to earn it. Another person's pain registers as an experience in the perceiver: empathy as forced symmetry, a bodily echo.

"Just think," Laz tells me. "Julian's *out there* somewhere."

Out there is a phrase that comes up frequently around camp. So

frequently, in fact, that one of the regular racers—a wiry old man
named "Frozen Ed" Furtaw (like Frozen Head, get it?), who runs in
sunset-orange camo tights—has self-published a book called *Tales
from* Out There: *The Barkley Marathons.* The book details each
year's comet trail of DNFs and includes an elaborate appendix list-
ing other atrociously difficult trail races and explaining why they're
not as hard.

"I was proud of Julian," I tell Laz. "It was dark and cold and he
could barely swallow his can of Ensure and he just put his head in
his hands and said: *Here I go.*"

Laz laughs. "How do you think he feels about that decision
now?"

It starts to rain. I make a nest in the back of my car. I type notes
for this essay. I watch an episode of *The Real World: Vegas* and then
turn it off, just as Steven and Trishelle are about to maybe hook up,
to conserve power for the next day and also because I don't want to
watch Steven and Trishelle hook up. I wanted her to hook up with
Frank. I try to sleep. I dream about the prison tunnel: it's flooding,
and I've just gotten a speeding ticket, and these two things are re-
lated in an important way I can't yet fathom. I'm awoken every once
in a while by the mournful call of bugle Taps, like the noises of a wild
animal echoing through the night.

Julian arrives back in camp around eight in the morning. He was
out for another twelve hours, but he only managed to reach two
books. There were a couple of hours lost, another couple spent lying
down, in the rain, waiting for first light. He is proud of himself for
going out, even though he didn't think he'd get far, and I am proud
of him too.

We join the others under the rain tent. Charlie Engle describes
what forced him back during his third loop. "Fell flat on my ass
going down Rat Jaw," he said. "Then I got up and fell again, got up
and fell again. That was pretty much it."

There's a nicely biblical logic to this story: it's the third time that really does the trick, seals the deal, breaks the back, what have you.

Laz asks whether Charlie enjoyed the prison section. Laz asks everyone about the prison section, the way you'd ask about your kid's poem: *Did you like it?*

Charlie says he did like it, very much. He says the guards were friendly enough to give him directions. "They were good ol' Southern boys, those guys," and I can tell from the way he says it that Charlie considers himself a good ol' Southern boy as well. "They told us: *Just make yer way up that there holler . . .* and then those California boys with me, they turn and say: *What the fuck is a holler?*"

"You should have told them," says Laz, "that in Tennessee a holler is when you want to get out but you can't."

"That's exactly what I said!" Charlie tells us. "I said: when you're standing barefoot on a red ant hill—that's a holler. The hill we're about to climb—that's a holler."

The rain is unrelenting. Laz doesn't think anyone will get the full hundred this year. There were some stellar first laps but no one seems strong enough now. People are speculating about whether anyone will even finish the Fun Run. There are only six runners left with a shot. If anyone can finish, everyone agrees, it will be Blake. Laz has never seen him quit.

Julian and I share a leg of chicken slathered in BBQ sauce. There are only two left on the grill. It's a miracle the fire hasn't gone out. The chicken's good, and cooked as promised, steaming in our mouths against the chilly air.

A guy named Zane, with whom Julian ran much of his first loop, tells us he saw several wild boars on the trails at night. Was he scared? He was. One got close enough to send him scurrying off the edge of a switchback, fighting stick in hand. Would a stick have helped? We all agree, probably not.

A woman clad in what looks like an all-body Windbreaker has packed a plastic bag of clothes. Laz explains that her husband is one of the six runners left. She's planning to meet him at the Lookout Tower. If he decides to drop, she'll hand him his dry clothes and escort him down the easy three-mile trail back into camp. If he decides to continue, she'll wish him luck as he prepares for another uphill climb—soaked in rainwater and pride, unable to take the dry clothes because accepting aid would get him disqualified.

"I hope she shows him the dry clothes *before* he makes up his mind," says Laz. "Choice is better that way."

The crowd stirs. There's a runner coming up the paved hill. Coming from this direction is a bad sign for someone on his third loop—it means he's dropping rather than finishing. People guess it's JB or Carl—*must be* JB or Carl, there aren't many guys still out—but after a moment Laz gasps.

"It's Blake," he says. "I recognize his walking poles."

Blake is soaked and shivering. "I'm close to hypothermia," he said. "I couldn't do it." He says that climbing Rat Jaw was like scrambling up a playground slide in roller skates, but otherwise he doesn't seem inclined to offer excuses. He says he was running with JB for a while but left him on Rat Jaw. "That's bad news for JB," says Laz, shaking his head. "He'll probably be back here soon."

Laz hands the bugle over. It's as if he can't bear to play Taps for Blake himself. He's clearly disappointed that Blake is out, but there's also a note of glee in his voice when he says: "You never know what'll happen around here." There's a thrill in the tension between controlling the race and recognizing it as something that will always disobey him. It approximates the tense pleasure of ultrarunning itself: the simultaneous exertion and ceding of power, controlling the body enough to make it run this thing but ultimately offering it to the uncontrollable vagaries of luck and endurance and conditions.

Doc Joe motions me over to the fire pit. "Hold this," he says, and shoves a large rectangle of aluminum siding in my direction. He balances a fallen tree branch against its edge to make a tepee over the fire, where the single remaining breast of chicken is crisping to a beautiful charred brown. "Blake's chicken," he explains. "I'll cover it with my body if I have to."

Why this sense of stakes and heroism? Of course I've been wondering the whole time: why do people *do* this, anyway? Whenever I pose the question directly, runners reply ironically: *I'm a masochist: I need somewhere to put my craziness; type A from birth,* etc. I begin to understand that joking about this question is not an evasion but rather an intrinsic part of answering it. Nobody has to answer this question seriously because they are already answering it seriously—with their bodies and their willpower and their pain. The body submits itself in earnest, in degradation and commitment, to what words can only speak of lightly. Maybe this is why so many ultrarunners are former addicts: they want to redeem the bodies they once punished, master the physical selves whose cravings they once served.

There is a gracefully frustrating tautology to this embodied testimony: *Why do I do it? I do it because it hurts so much and I'm still willing to do it.* The sheer ferocity of the effort implies that the effort is somehow worth it. This is purpose by implication rather than direct articulation. Laz says: "No one has to ask them why they're out here; they all know."

It would be easy to fix upon any number of possible purposes: conquering the body, fellowship in pain, but it *feels* more like significance dwells in concentric circles of labor around an empty center—commitment to an impetus that resists fixity or labels. The persistence of "why" is the point: the elusive horizon of an unanswerable question, the conceptual equivalent of an unrunnable race.

But: how does the race turn out?

Turns out JB, Jonboy, a relatively new kid on the starting block, the returning champion's best support crew, manages to pull off a surprising victory. Which makes the fifth paragraph of this essay a lie: the race has nine finishers now. I get this news as a text message from Julian, who found out from Twitter. We're both driving home on separate highways. My immediate thought is: *shit*. I wasn't planning to focus on JB as a central character in my essay—he hadn't seemed like one of the strongest personalities or contenders at camp—but now I know I'll have to turn him into a story too.

This is what Barkley specializes in, right? It swallows the story you imagined and hands you another one. Blake and Carl—both strong after their second loops, two of my chosen figures of interest—didn't even finish the Fun Run.

Now everyone goes home. Carl will go back to his machine shop in Atlanta. Blake will help his daughter train for the trials. John Price will return to his retirement and his man-wagon. Laz, I discover, will return to his position as assistant coach for the boy's basketball team at Cascade High School, down the highway in Wartrace.

One of the most compelling inquiries into the question of *why*—to my mind, at least—is really an inquiry around the question, and it lies in a tale of temporary madness: AT's frightening account of his fifth-loop "crisis of purpose" back in 2004.

By "crisis of purpose," he means: "losing my mind in the full definition of the phrase," a relatively unsurprising condition, given circumstances. He's not alone in this experience. Brett Maune describes hallucinating a band of helpful Indians at the end of his three-day run of the John Muir Trail:

> They watched over me while I slept and I would chat with them briefly every time I awoke. They were very considerate and even helped me pack everything when I was ready to resume hiking. I hope this does not count as aid!

AT describes wandering without any clear sense of how he'd gotten there or what he was meant to be doing: "The Barkley would be forgotten for minutes on end although the premise lingered. I HAD to get to the Garden Spot, for . . . *why*? Was there someone there?"

His amnesia captures the endeavor in its starkest terms: premise without motivation, hardship without context. It was not without flashes of wonder:

> I stood in a shin-deep puddle for about an hour—squishing the mud in and out of my shoes . . . I walked down to Coffin Springs (the first water drop). I sat and poured gallon after gallon of fresh water into my shoes . . . I inspected the painted trees, marking the park boundary; sometimes walking well into the woods just to look at some paint on a tree.

In a sense, Barkley does precisely this: forces its runners into an appreciation of what they might not otherwise have known or noticed—the ache in their quads when they have been punished beyond all reasonable measure, fatigue pulling the body's puppet strings inexorably downward, the mind gone numb and glassy from pain.

By the end of AT's account, the facet of Barkley deemed most brutally taxing, that sinister and sacred "self-sufficiency," has become an inexplicable miracle:

> When it cooled off, I had a long-sleeve shirt. When I got hungry, I had food. When it got dark, I had a light. I thought: *Wow, isn't it strange that I have all this perfect stuff, just when I need it?*

This is benevolence as surprise, evidence of a grace beyond the self that has, of course, come *from* the self—the same self that loaded the fanny pack hours before, whose role has been obscured by bone-weary delusion. So it goes. One morning a man blows a conch shell, and two days later—still answering the call of that conch, another man finds all he needs strapped to his own body, where he can neither expect nor explain it.

IN DEFENSE
⁚ OF SACCHARIN(E) ⁚

Human speech is like a cracked pot on which we beat out
rhythms for bears to dance to when we are striving to make
music that will wring tears from the stars.
— GUSTAVE FLAUBERT, *Madame Bovary*

Saccharine is our sweetest word for fear: the fear of too much sentiment, too much taste. When we hear *saccharin*, we think of cancer:
too many cells congealing in the body. When we hear *saccharine*,
we think of language that has shamed us, netted our hearts in trite
articulations: words repeated too many times for cheap effect, re-
cycled ad nauseam. *Ad nauseam:* we are glutted with sweet to the
point of sickness.

Some Ideas about the Thing: I have an entire trash can in my kitchen
full of empty artificial sweetener packets. It's small. It's not that
small. I keep it next to the stove, out of sight from visitors.

If *sentimentality* is the word people use to insult emotion—in its
simplified, degraded, and indulgent forms—then "saccharine" is the
word they use to insult sentimentality. It traces back to the Sanskrit
sarkara, meaning "gravel" or "grit." It meant "like sugar" until the
nineteenth century, when it started to mean "too much." It started
as a concept but turned into a danger. Scientists fed their lab rats
loads of saccharin and then they started getting bladder tumors.

My college roommate took a photograph of me the night before
a physics final during our sophomore year. In this photo, I am lying
on my bed. She has piled empty cans and bottles all over my body to

show how much Diet Coke I'd consumed that day. You can only see my face and hands. Everything else is covered.

The Thing Itself: is just a powder, so light that a little bit drifts onto my counter each time I tear open another packet. Gravel or grit— something pounded to dust.

When I was young, I lived in a house with windows for walls. During the long days of summer, I sat on our deck and watched blue jays fly into the glass, knock themselves out, drop stone-like to the redwood planks below. Mostly they were trying to get in but sometimes— and this was worse to watch—they'd gotten trapped inside and were trying to get out again. I told my mother that the birds mistook our windows for the surface of the sky. She took my hand and showed me a bush growing just beyond our front door. She said the birds got drunk on its berries, which were orange like rust stains and full of sugar. She said the birds couldn't stop eating them. They got strange and woozy. That's why they kept on crashing.

I didn't know about fermentation back then but I did know about sweetness, its shameful thrall. I knew things about those birds, even as a child: the glass sky was flatter and harder than they imagined, and through it they could see a world it wouldn't let them reach.

When I was eight years old, my parents gave me a glass of wine at a dinner party. It was two-hundred-dollar wine but I didn't know that. I snuck into the kitchen and dumped in a spoonful of sugar to make it taste better. I felt ashamed of this, but didn't know why. I couldn't think of how to defend myself, or why I would need to.

In *Madame Bovary*, Félicité the maid is always scuttling away from some new abuse at the hands of her self-involved mistress. She seeks sweetness as consolation: "since Madame always left the key in the sideboard, Félicité took a small supply of sugar every night and ate it when she was all alone in her bed, after she had said her prayers."

How could sugar still be necessary after prayer? It offers salve to the physical body, immediate comfort, something the flesh can trust while the spirit is being patient. Think of the sadness of two women living in the same house, both hungry for stolen increments of different pleasures—text and lust and sugar—both keeping these pleasures secret because they are ashamed to admit their hungers.

I know I'd find something to steal from Emma's sideboard, if given the chance. I've always tucked indulgences away from others' sight. I spent years bending over my lattes so that nobody could see how many packets of aspartame I'd shaken into them.

I hated *Madame Bovary* when I was sixteen, and its heroine too. I thought they were too emotional, novel and protagonist alike, too overt with their passions. But I love it now—the book, if not its heroine. I enjoy analyzing her melodrama, even if I haven't forgiven her for indulging it. I also want it for myself. I always have: those highs and lows of feeling, everything turned superlative. I've lifted emotional blueprints from Emma just like she lifted them from books of her own. The same hunger sends us to prayer and sugar and sweetener and text: the rush of comfort that comes from quick taste, the body suddenly filled with a sensation beyond itself—foreign and seductive.

Sentimentality is an accusation leveled against unearned emotion. Oscar Wilde summed up the indignation: "A sentimentalist is simply one who desires to have the luxury of an emotion without paying for it." Artificial sweeteners grant the same intensity—sweeter than sugar itself—without the price: no tax of calories. They offer the shell of sugar without its substance; this feels miraculous and hideous at once.

This isn't to say that sweeteners are the same as sentimentality—or even a perfect symbol for it—but simply to suggest that a similar fear is operative in these different spheres of taste. Both terms describe sweetness—emotion or taste—that feels shallow, exaggerated or undeserved, ultimately unreal. The gut reacts toward and against, seeking a vocabulary to contain excess, to name and accuse and banish it: too much sentiment, unmediated by nuance; too much sweet, undisciplined by restraint. The hunger for unmitigated and uncomplicated sensation carries on its tongue an unspoken shame. "You are a little soul carrying around a corpse," Epicetus once said. The body is a monstrous thing that turns the soul grotesque, and that sentimental craving for a quick fix of feeling, or sudden rush of sweet, feels like the emotional equivalent of that cumbersome luggage—corporeal and base—an embarrassing set of desires that our ethereal, higher selves have to lug around. Melodrama is something to binge on: cupcakes in the closet.

Texts are dispatched by the clean guillotine strokes of these accusatory words: saccharine, syrupy, sentimental. We dismiss sentimentality in order to construct ourselves as arbiters of artistry and subtlety, so sensitive we don't need the same crude quantities of feeling—those blunt surfaces, baggy corpses. We will subsist more delicately, we say. We will subsist on less.

In a review called "Tides of Treacle," James Wood describes the texture of a novelist's sentimentality: "Again and again, one catches [her] in the process of exaggerating a good idea, of adding sugar to a mixture already sweet enough." In a song called "Sentimental Movie," Axl Rose croons: "I'm peeking on for some pain," watching and addressing a beloved who is shooting up to shut pain down: "put on a pad on your vein." But even Guns N' Roses—the band that gave us Slash ripping his ferocious guitar solo on the open plains—shares a disdain for sentimentality, "peeking on" at feelings that are ultimately hollow: "This ain't no Sentimental Movie / Where dreams collect like dust." Sentimentality inflates a feeling into something that can't sustain itself—a dream shape—that ultimately flakes off into dust, grit or gravel, useless remains.

In "What Is Wrong with Sentimentality?," philosopher Mark Jefferson describes it as "an emotional indulgence that involves misrepresenting the world," but also specifies its mode of misrepresentation ("a simplistic appraisal") and its potential consequences: "a direct impairment to the moral vision taken of its subject." The danger of sentimentality is that it might distort emotions to excuse or sustain societal evils, and Jefferson stresses that it is "not

something that simply befalls people." He speaks of sentimental-
ists as "hosts" complicit in harboring their own indulgent feelings:
"we don't know . . . why it is that certain emotion types are more
likely hosts for it than others." His rhetoric summons the image of
a worm coiled in our stomachs, waiting for whatever melodrama we
find to feed it. I have recurring dreams about parasites, alien creatures that hatch from eggs beneath my skin, and I imagine Jefferson
showing up inside them, shying away as I explain my condition: *I've
got a bad case of the sentimentals.*

Fellow philosopher Michael Tanner also frames sentimentality
in terms of contagion. He called it a "disease of the feelings," as if we
could find its ungainly tumors of excess inside of us, metastasizing
like cells inside a lab rat's bladder. Susan Sontag talks about sentimentality like internal machinery: "You can't imagine how tiring it
is. That double-membraned organ of nostalgia, pumping the tears
in. Pumping them out."

In a 1979 op-ed called "In Defense of Sentimentality," John
Irving examines the legacy of Dickens's *A Christmas Carol,* stressing
the importance of what he calls "Christmas risks": earnest attempts
to articulate pathos without cloaking it in cleverness or wit.

In another "In Defense of Sentimentality," philosopher Robert
Solomon responds to thinkers like Jefferson and Tanner, teas-
ing out the differences between distinct critiques of sentimentality that often get lumped into a single campaign. Is the problem of
sentimentality primarily ethical or aesthetic? Solomon paraphrases
Tanner's argument that "sentimental people indulge their feelings instead of doing what should be done" and cites the example
of Nazi commander Rudolf Hoess, who wept at an opera staged
by concentration camp prisoners. Perhaps this wasn't simply ironic
but actually causal: His sentimental experience was an escape valve
releasing pressure that should have been troubling his conscience.

While its moral critics attack sentimentality because it accords
an undue agency to emotions—distracting us from conceptually rig-
orous or logistically tenable ethics—its aesthetic opponents attack

sentimentality from another direction, claiming it does our emotions a disservice by flattening them into hyperbole or simplicity. Wallace Stevens called sentimentality a "failure of feeling," but his syntax is ambiguous: does he mean that we've failed our feelings or that they've failed us?

This ambiguity seems to circle back to Solomon's distinction. Is the idea that feelings are not enough, that they will fail us if we rely on them too exclusively (for ethical decisions) or milk their excessive impact too shamelessly (for aesthetic value)? Or is the idea that our language is often not enough for feelings themselves, that sentimentality forces them into artificial vessels or cheap bulk-good volumes? Are there right and wrong ways to experience emotion in response to aesthetic work? On the one hand, an overly simple response that can be ethically problematic; and on the other hand, a more nuanced response—more attentive to the world outside the text—that can be ethically productive?

If these are the array of charges implicitly being leveled each time somebody uses the word *sentimentality* as a derogatory shortcut, then it seems they need to be specified: At what volume does feeling become sentimental? How obliquely does feeling need to be rendered so it can be saved from itself? How do we distinguish between pathos and melodrama? Too often, I think, there is the sense that we *just know*. Well I don't.

In Stevens's poem "The Revolutionists Stop for Orangeade," a group of guerrilla soldiers stand "flat-ribbed and big-bagged" in the glare of noon. Their captains tell them not to sing in the sun, but they imagine singing anyway: "a song of serpent-kin, / Necks among the thousand leaves, / Tongues around the fruit." The poem imagines trivial aesthetics amid wreckage, the taste of something simple and sweet asserting itself into a complicated history. This taste is delivered by a serpent—the original agent of the fall, the first sweet fruit—but one senses also a relishing, a celebration. First the orangeade, then the rebellion. First the bad singing, then the good fight. And what if the flavor of orange is mimicry? What if the tongues have found false fruit? What if the words of the song aren't true? The poem dares to make a case for the refuge of artificiality: "There is no pith in music / Except in something false."

A memory: I'm drinking Jim Beam in a bar three blocks off Bourbon Street. I'm drinking this whiskey because I'd like to become a different version of myself. This desire is directed toward the poet I've recently fallen in love with, who is drinking his own tumbler of the same brand. Jim shares its name and we joke about what this means for his destiny. When he isn't making jokes, he's talking about the role of the epic in our time. He talks about wanting poetry to tackle the grand sweep of human events. He also sometimes talks about living in purgatory, inside the curse of his life. He tells me he used to know a serial killer.

"I mean," he says, "it's not like I knew him that well."

You have to understand a few things about my relationship with Jim. He was darkness and I was light. I was innocence and he was experience. (He was big-time into Blake.) I wrote fiction and he wrote poetry. I lived in what he called "the real world" and he didn't, quite. I was younger than I'd told him. He wasn't exactly old, but he was just coming out of a relationship with a woman who'd gotten cervical cancer that he hadn't been able to cure. This added years. The woman was also vaguely superhuman, or so he claimed. She made him feel a kind of "total emotion" he hadn't felt since. She'd once channeled the spirit of James Merrill outside a donut shop in rural Wyoming. She was lots of things I'd never be.

So this serial killer worked the after-party hours at a pizza place near Jim's college. He was a big black guy, a real whiz with the rolling slicer and a friendly face to all. He kept working his shift right up until they found a body on his property, and then another, and then a third.

"It's just strange to know you were that close to total evil," Jim says.

I think about that for a moment: Jim's pride at brushing against darkness, my pride at sleeping with someone who'd brushed against darkness like that.

Then I think about this: how I'd like a different drink than what I'm drinking. I am one of the revolutionists, thirsty for orangeade by the side of the road. I want one of those bright plastic mugs they drink from on Bourbon Street, full of frozen daiquiris that taste like they're trying to trump their namesake fruits. My sister-in-law calls these artificial flavors "Obsequious Watermelon," "Obsequious Apple," "Obsequious Banana." These drinks are working overtime to grant their favors.

Obsequious seems right: attempting to win favor by flattery. Isn't this the problem of saccharine literature? That it strokes the ego of our sentimental selves? That we're flattered when something illuminates our capacity to feel? That this satisfaction replaces genuine emotional response?

I turn to Jim, find a way to phrase my desire: "I want to drink something sweet."

We go in search of drinks called Twisters and Hurricanes. Their ridiculous names will feel like ghosts, years later, once the levees break and the city floods.

It matters to me that New Orleans no longer exists as it once did, when I shared it with a man who no longer exists to me as he used to. Perhaps this is nothing more than a pathetic fallacy: the loss of love writ large, demanding the submersion of an entire city. But why is it that my memories offer me back to myself in my most trivial moments? Why do I hunger for significant barometers but find myself tethered to banality instead?

I remember demanding a Hurricane and feeling ashamed for wanting one. I remember talking about drinks rather than serial killers. I remember secretly dismissing phrases like "total evil" and "grand sweep of human events" and "total emotion," because I felt they were too large and too vague to do much good. But I was also afraid of those phrases. I remember that too.

In a reconstructed laboratory somewhere in downtown Baltimore, two mannequins are having an argument: "It makes my blood boil to see the lies of that scoundrel Fahlberg!" one says, then interrupts his own recorded self: "Pardon my outburst. I am Dr. Ira Remsen."

The stiff-limbed figure of Constantin Fahlberg defends himself quickly, a taped voice clogged with heavy Russian inflections: "He didn't have anything to do with the manufacturing process!" He jerks his arm to signify emotion.

These automatons are fighting about the origins of Sweet'N Low. It's fitting that their feelings have been rendered with such robotic strokes, imitating the discovery of an imitation: saccharin (né cameorthobezoyl sulfamide.) They both discovered the thing, or think they did. It happened in Remsen's lab, but it was Fahlberg's sleuth-work. Remsen took the credit for the paper. Fahlberg took the profits on the patent. It was like this:

One day Fahlberg was working with coal tar and got some chemicals on his sleeve. That night, his bread tasted sweeter than usual. He got curious. He went back to the lab and started tasting residues on white coats, sampling chemicals straight from their tubes. These were unsafe lab practices, made possible by unsanitary conditions. But he managed to discover a kind of sugar the body refused to metabolize. At last, we would be able to glut ourselves on pleasure without finding its residue lodged in our expanding girth.

This is part of what we disdain about sweeteners, the fact that we can taste without consequences. Our capitalist ethos loves a certain kind of inscription—insisting we can read tallies of sloth and discipline inscribed across the body itself—and artificial sweeteners threaten this legibility. They offer a way to cheat the arithmetic of indulgence and bodily consequence, just like sentimentality offers feeling without the price of complication. As Wilde said: *the luxury of an emotion without paying for it.* It's a kind of Horatio Alger–bootstrap ethos in our aesthetic economy: you need to *earn* your reactions to art, not simply collect easy sentiment handed out like welfare.

How do we earn? By parsing figurative opacity, close-reading metaphor, tracking nuances of character, historicizing in terms of print history and social history and institutional history and trans-oceanic history and every other kind of history we can think of. We think we should have to work in order to feel. We want to have our cake resist us; and then we want to eat it, too.

We're disgusted when anything comes too easily. But also greedy. Some women describe heaven as a place where food doesn't have calories. Frank Bidart's poem "Ellen West" begins with an anorexic woman confessing "heaven / would be dying on a bed of vanilla ice cream." She'd get the exquisite freedom of indulgence without bodily consequence—no price to pay in fat or weight or presence because she'd already be dead. And now we have this heaven here on earth, death in life: sweeteners liberate our bodies from the sins of our mouths.

Some Important Dates in the History of Artificial Sugar:

1879—In Remsen's Baltimore lab, Constantin Fahlberg forgets to wash his hands. He finds saccharin.

1937—Michael Sveda tastes something sweet on the end of his cigarette at the University of Illinois. This is cyclamate.

1965—James Schlatter licks some amino acids off his fingertips. Aspartame!

1976—An assistant researcher at the Tate & Lyle sugar company misunderstands directions, tastes instead of tests, discovers sucralose.

The scientists behind our major artificial sweeteners compose a motley crew of dilettantes, a catalog of Ways-to-Fuck-Up-in-the-Lab. These aren't the Alexander Flemings of our scientific mythologies, our accidental heroes. They stumble onto things we're not sure we wanted found. They aren't the guys we're proud of.

So many times during the course of this essay I have risen from my computer to dump small blue packets of Equal into a fresh cup of tea. The residue of their powder makes a fine silt over my counters. I

am like Fahlberg or Sveda, always tasting sweet where I don't expect
to find it: on my wine glasses and my vegetable knives, the edges of
my ballpoint pens.

Donald Barthelme's story "Wrack" is about a man who disavows
everything he owns: a dressing gown, a woman's shoe, a single slice
of salami sandwiched by two fat mattresses. "You mean to say that
you think *I* would own a bonbon dish?" he asks an undisclosed ap-
praiser. "A sterling-silver or whatever it is bonbon dish? You're mad."

One item that he *doesn't* immediately disavow is this: a hundred-
pound sack of saccharin. I was delighted to read this. Finally! An
owning. But the defense is abandoned almost immediately: the man
explains his sack by way of a "condition" that forbids the intake of
sugar. He backs away from the specter of the sweet sack: "I just remember, I put sugar in my coffee, at breakfast . . . it was definitely
sugar. Granulated. So the sack of saccharin is definitely not mine."
We watch a character define himself entirely through what he will
not claim.

If I could choose one item from my entire apartment, what
would I disown? It might be my trash can full of ripped paper packets, which might mean that this pile of packets is my most honest
expression of self.

Saccharin manages to function as a pretty ubiquitous locus of dis-
avowal. A *New Yorker* "Talk of the Town" from 1937 describes a
woman who finds a tiny platinum box at Saks but can't figure out
its purpose:

> "That?" the [sales]girl said. "Why, that's used for saccharin. Or
> for birdseed." She thought for a moment or so, seemingly a little
> startled by her own explanation, then repeated, more firmly, "Or
> for birdseed."

It's okay to feed the birds but not to glut ourselves, at least
on something so tacky. One imagines the box as a secret tool of

indulgence: a kind of culinary vessel for slumming it or else the deliciously clandestine machinery of classier mischief, some high-society debutante sniffing Sweet'N Low like coke. What's sketched by these other lines of clean white powder? The shamefully legible notes of our least complicated desires.

Jim and I relocate to Bourbon Street, where we don't drink whiskey. We take bright pink shots from test tubes while middle-aged revelers dance through our peripheral vision. I pull out some praline I bought that afternoon while he walked along the river alone. He needed a break from me, he said, but not unkindly.

We have ongoing arguments about the expression of sentiment. These arguments are ostensibly aesthetic, but really they are personal, the same old fights that couples who don't write poetry or fiction have every single day, yelling across molded aspic salads: *You say too much about your feelings. You don't say enough. When you speak, it's in the wrong language.*

Jim was the one who told me that my emotional life made him dangle his stethoscope like a snake charmer: my moods weren't hard to see but they were hard to read, and even harder to diagnose. It was ostensibly a complaint, but I think he liked his metaphor, and liked that our moments of distance were subtle enough to require this kind of formulation.

Meaning that I was a complex creature and so was he; that he became even more complex in his attempt to bridge the gap between our complexities; that he could create a complicated image to house this complex of complications. This is how writers fall in love: they feel complicated together and then they talk about it.

Figurative language often delivers us to the saccharine, drawing from its familiar grab-bag of tear-jerker props ("voice like honey," "porcelain skin," "waterfall of tears"), but it can also offer an escape hatch out of the predictability of sentiment. Metaphors are tiny saviors leading the way out of sentimentality, small disciples of Pound, urging "Say it new! Say it new!" It's hard for emotion to feel flat if its language is suitably novel, to feel excessive if its rendering is suitably opaque. Metaphors translate emotion into surprising and sublime language, but they also help us deflect and diffuse the glare of revelation. Stevens describes this shyness: "The motive for metaphor, shrinking from / The weight of primary noon, / The ABC of being."

Jim was afraid to speak in simple language—the ABC of being— so he spoke about cobras instead. This was not cowardice exactly, but rather a distaste for the bald and unexciting phraseology of relationships: the kind of thing that *anyone* might say to his girlfriend, rather than the particular thing that Jim could say to me.

What do we flee when we retreat into metaphor? What scares us about primary noon? Kundera claims that "kitsch moves us to tears for ourselves, for the banality of what we think and feel," and I think our fixation with complication and opaque figuration has something to do with an abiding sense of this banality, creeping constantly around the edges of our lives and language. Perhaps if we say it straight, we suspect, if we express our sentiments too excessively or too directly, we'll find we're nothing but banal.

There are several fears inscribed in this suspicion: not simply about melodrama or simplicity but about commonality, the fear that our feelings will resemble everyone else's. This is why we want to dismiss sentimentality, to assert instead that our emotional responses are more sophisticated than other people's, that our aesthetic sensibilities testify, iceberg style, to an entire landscape of interior depth.

When they released NutraSweet in the 1980s, GD Searle & Co. knew that they needed an icon to assert novelty and familiarity at once. They were thinking basic shapes, vague connotations, comfort colors. In a way, they were looking for the opposite of Stevens's motivated metaphor. They wanted a symbol that could descend into the belly of the "primary," eschew complication and mystery in favor of assurance.

Searle hired two people who hadn't—by their own report— tasted sugar in a decade. They were wary of choosing an image that was too sugary, too obviously rummaged from an old grab bag of tropes. The *New Yorker* quotes one of them on this dilemma:

"We'd have a meeting with the agency people, and someone would say, 'What about hearts? Hearts are friendly. Hearts are sweet' . . . They were talking about things that would have been absolutely saccharine."

Even here, at its birthplace, saccharin disavows its namesake. It wants to protest the charge of being too much itself.

The Internet is full of saccharin-savvy doomsday prophets. They've got the dirt on cancer and FDA cover-ups. Their counterparts are scarcer. Saccharin-nut blogger Katie Kinker has this to say about our modern world:

Without artificial sweeteners, what would life be like today? Would their [sic] be tastey [sic] diet drinks, fruit juice drinks, chewing gum etc.? There wouldn't be any pink or blue packets to dump into your iced tea. Things would be bland, and honestly, it is hard to imagine a society without artificial sweeteners. They are everywhere! Thank goodness for serendipity!

Katie achieves an almost perfect apotheosis of poor taste and saccharine attachments. If she ever found a tiny platinum box, she'd be tacky enough to load it up with Sweet'N Low. She probably reads Harlequin romance novels and cries at movies about dogs rescuing their injured owners. She is the quintessential object of a disdain I project onto some faceless saccharin(e)-hating other: she's got an underdeveloped palate, an overdeveloped appetite, and an oversized heart.

I am trying to remember how I first learned that sentimentality was something I should be running away from. Even the end of the world starts with a saccharine text. Witness the Book of Revelation, where John is warned of an apocalyptic book. He is told: "It will be as sweet as honey in your mouth." He is told: "It will make your stomach bitter."

I think my fear might trace back to the *Harvard Advocate*, a literary magazine whose clapboard house was my nursery through most of college. I spent countless nights smoking cigarettes in a wood-paneled sanctum and bantering with other smokers about the terrible clichés we found in our submissions, about half of which we'd written ourselves.

Last night, I sat at my computer and Googled "Harvard Advocate + melodrama," thinking I would find some collection of scathing reviews we'd published in the magazine, accusations steeped in irony and leveled against art that dared to feel anything too unabashedly. I'd find some record of our collective taste proclaiming itself, a dismissal of shameless sentiment.

In the end, I found only one entry. It was a quote from one of my own stories:

> She imagined him as an executioner during childhood, probably only of bugs, possibly a few small or particularly deserving mammals. She guessed that he still lay awake some nights, haunted by the memory of these acts. He would never say haunted, though, she was sure of that. He seemed like the type to find that kind of melodrama unseemly.

Turns out *I* was the one preoccupied with the unseemliness of melodrama. I was just like the woman I'd written: always imagining that others had a problem with sentimentality because I couldn't figure out the problem I had with it myself.

When I packed off for the Iowa Writers' Workshop, I had a set of vague ideas about what I wanted to be writing. I wanted to write stories that were smart and funny and ruthless but I had no idea what they'd be about. I knew I didn't want to write anything sentimental. My primary rudder was a morbid fear of anything too tender, too touchy-feely. So I created characters who hated themselves and disavowed pretty much everything around them. One of the first stories I wrote at the Workshop was about a girl named Sophie, whom I'd bequeathed with abysmal self-esteem and a slew of circumstances to justify it.

In response to my piece, one guy wrote: "I know someone's going to want to kick me in the balls for saying this, but there are times when it seems like the author is just lining up Sophie's misfortunes. She has a facial deformity that has crippled her self-esteem, she is sexually assaulted, guys don't like her, she may have an eating disorder, and she's a transfer student. Does anything ever go right for Sophie?"

It was a fair point. Sophie hated herself because I hated her too. I resented her for coaxing me into writing such a melodramatic story. I hated myself for making her hate herself so much.

I wasn't the only one who felt this way. Another guy's critique began like this: "I should start by saying that I did not find any of the characters likable at all . . . I had to follow characters I had trouble caring about while they did things I had trouble believing they cared about." It was true: I'd been wary of giving Sophie much agency or investment. I knew the events of her story hovered at the brink of melodrama, and I feared that if I let her do anything, she might fling herself over the edge. So I wrote her tale in language described as a "passive voice epidemic"—an accusation I still describe passively, even in retrospect.

My fear of too much emotion—and my secondary fear of this fear—had joined forces to yield an embittered hybrid. I had somehow managed to weave the failures of sentimentality and anti-sentimentality into a single story, summoned an exaggerated string of tragedies and used them to make sure everybody felt nothing.

The line between pathos and melodrama becomes a question of mechanism: If the tropes are too easy, the narrative too predictably mannered, the sentiments exaggerated for the sake of emotional manipulation, the language cloying rather than fresh—all these cheapen the eliciting of emotion. Sentimentality describes the moment when emotion becomes a prop to bolster the affective egos of everyone involved. "Kitsch causes two tears to flow in quick succession," Kundera observes. "The first tear says: how nice to see children running on the grass! The second tear says: How nice to be moved, together with all mankind, by children running on the grass."

This is truly the obsequious fruit of child-sized pastorals—an image offering itself too effusively, charming us into submission by coaxing out the vision of ourselves we'd most like to see. Our tears become trophies and emblems of our compassion.

But doesn't anti-sentimentality simply offer an inversion of that same affective ego boost? We reject sentimentality to sharpen a sense of ourselves as True Feelers, arbiters of complication and actual emotion. The anti-sentimental stance is still a mode of identity ratification, arrows flying instead of tears flowing, still a way to make a point about perceptive capacity: an assertion about discernment rather than empathy. It's self-righteousness by way of dismissal: a kind of masturbatory double negative.

Even if there's nothing aesthetically redeemable in the eliciting of the prepackaged double-tiered (teared) response that Kundrea describes, does it have some other value? How do we account for the pleasure people take in trashy romances or tearjerker films? What good is this mass eliciting of feeling? If it causes pleasure, isn't there something to respect in that—or do we plead false consciousness and argue otherwise? Do we insist that better artwork can elicit a better kind of feeling—more expansive, supple, ethical?

Even melodrama can carry someone across the gulf between his life and the lives of others. A terrible TV movie about addiction can still make someone feel for the addict—no matter how general this addict, how archetypal or paradigmatic, no matter how trite the plot twists, how shameful the puppetry of heart strings. Bad movies and bad writing and easy clichés still manage to make us feel things toward each other. Part of me is disgusted by this. Part of me celebrates it.

I once spent an hour and a half listening to Buffy Sainte-Marie on repeat: "For better your pain, than be caught on Co'dine . . . An' it's real, an' it's real, one more time." Co'dine puts a pad on the vein, and the song rips it off—*peeking on for some pain* instead of gauzing over it. It's a familiar tension between feeling something and repressing it; facing it, or refusing to. But listening to the song on repeat—me with my cigarettes, with my parasitic sorrow—dissolves that familiar binary. Indulging in the sadness of that song became an anesthetic in its own right, sentiment absorbed like a drug, a way to feel one simple note over and over again—instead of whatever mess was waiting for me once the music had quieted.

Now Jim and I are running through the cobblestone alleys of the French Quarter. Pastel paint peeling off walls shows the pastel snakeskins of older walls beneath. I'm riding piggyback. We're both screaming, because we are alive and in New Orleans and incredibly drunk and also—though we wear this knowledge lightly—in love with the person we're riding (in my case) or the person who is riding us (in his). We might have had different ideas about *how* to get drunk, but now there's nothing left to dispute. This is sweet. It asks no questions of us. We ask no questions in reply.

After breaking my heart, a poet (another poet!) wrote in one of his poems: "We drank coffee with so much cream we tasted only cream." I wondered if that had been our downfall. Maybe it has always been my downfall: too much cream; too much sweetener in my coffee.

Perhaps I let myself believe too easily or fully in the surface of joy without attending to the complications of its underbelly. Perhaps this is why I've broken up with so many men after the initial flush of love gives way to something else. Perhaps I've committed myself too absolutely to honeymoons to reckon with their aftermath. I have never been "sweetie" or "honey" to anyone. Whenever some boyfriend called me "sweet," it made me nervous: was I nothing more? It seemed so limited, seemed to state conclusively that something was lacking or wrong.

Honeymoon means days that are too sweet to last, to be real or deep in the ways we are accustomed to understanding depth or reality—in terms of nuance and continuity, the inevitable chiaroscuro of highs and lows. The state of being intoxicated by the taste of honey—cloying, consuming—is juxtaposed as innocence against the harder task of lasting human relation. But is this the whole sad truth of sweetness? Its saturation point? Its ceiling?

How can I express my faith that there is something profound in the single note of honey itself? In our uncomplicated capacity for rapture, the ability to find our whole selves moved by something infinitely simple? I'm not sure how to say it right, with the kind of language that would be sentimental enough to support its point but not too sentimental to damn it.

Maybe I'm still talking to the poet, long after he stopped talking to me. Maybe I'm writing to justify myself, or else surrender completely: *I could make you another cup of coffee, I swear! I could make this one without so much cream—or else we could keep on drinking cream forever!* Maybe that poet wasn't even writing about me at all.

"You're so vain," sang Carly Simon. "You probably think this song is about you."

"Let's be honest," said Warren Beatty. "That song was about me."

When we criticize sentimentality, perhaps part of what we fear is the possibility that it allows us to usurp the texts we read, insert ourselves and our emotional needs too aggressively into their narratives, clog their situations and their syntax with our tears. Which brings us back to the danger that we're mainly crying for ourselves, or at least to feel ourselves cry.

Mark Jefferson claims that sentimentality involves a choice. His theory holds that people choose to engage in distorted representations of reality so they can feel things in response. He describes sentimentality as a particular kind of inherited distortion, a "fiction of innocence" that demands complementary fictions of villainy, and that these fictions create a "moral climate that will sanction crude antipathy and its active expression." I agree that sentimentality permits these fictions, but I don't think these fictions always create the kind of moral climate he fears, nor do they necessitate the unequivocally reductive aesthetic response ("crude antipathy") assumed by his argument.

I think sometimes sentimentality inspires antipathy and sometimes it doesn't; sometimes this antipathy is useful and sometimes it isn't; sometimes compassion gets summoned instead. I think the presence of choice—in our responses to sentimental fiction—also suggests the possibility of more self-aware reception: we can let ourselves feel without letting those feelings stand unexamined.

The truth is, I resist something in sentimentality too. I'm afraid of its inflated gestures and broken promises. But I'm just as afraid of what happens when we run away from it: jadedness, irony, chill. I'm not immune to the siren call of either pole. My own work was once called "cold fiction," which I don't think was wrong. I made Sophie suffer but I didn't make her care about it. I've caught myself in all stages of the sentimental guilt/indulgence cycle: clutching tragedy and then fleeing its ramifications; taking refuge in feelings gone molten or frozen in compensation.

I'm not the first voice to call for sentimentality in the wake of postmodern irony. There's a chorus. There's been a chorus for years. Once upon a time, it was directed by David Foster Wallace. Now it's directed by his ghost. "An ironist in an AA meeting is a witch in church," he wrote in *Infinite Jest*, and for him the deeply earnest clichés of recovery represented one vector of literary possibility: the recuperated sentimentality of "single-entendre" writing, big crude crayon-drawing feelings that could actually render us porous to one another—clichés that he positioned inside the infinitely complicated landscape of his imagined worlds. He was searching for literature that could make our "heads throb heartlike," that could hold feeling and its questioning at once.

I believe in the possibility of this heartlike throbbing. I believe in the possibility of Christmas risks. I believe in an interrogated sentimentality that doesn't allow its distortions to be inherited so easily. I want to make a case for the value of that moment when we feel sentimentality punctured—when we feel its flatness revealed, that sense of a vista splitting open or opening out. Something useful happens in that moment of breakage. After the sugar high, always, dwells a sharpened sense of everything not sweet. If the saccharine offers some undiluted spell of feeling—oversimplified and unabashedly fictive—then perhaps its value lies in the process of emerging from its thrall: that sense of unmasking, that sense of guilt. We try to wring tears from the stars but can't ever quite forget the cracked kettles of our attempts, or the ways our music is always broken.

I want us to feel swollen by sentimentality and then hurt by it, betrayed by its flatness, wounded by the hard glass surface of its sky. This is one way to approach Stevens's primary noon. We crash into wonder—fling ourselves upon simplicity—so it can render us heavy and senseless, deliver us finally to the ground.

❖ FOG COUNT ❖

It's early morning and I'm hunting for quarters. Downtown Fayetteville is quiet and full of stately stone buildings: mining money, probably. We're in the heart of coal country. The corner diner isn't open yet. The "Only Creole Restaurant in West Virginia" isn't open yet. City Hall isn't open yet. Its window holds a flier raising money to build a treehouse for a girl named Izzy.

I'm looking for quarters because I'm headed to prison. I've been told they will be useful there. I'm going to see a man named Charlie Engle, with whom I've been corresponding for the past nine months. He has promised that if I bring quarters we can binge on junk food from the vending machines while we talk. Visiting hours are 8 to 3. It makes me nervous to think about talking from 8 to 3. I'm afraid I'll forget all my questions or that my questions are wrong anyway. I'm plotting my meals in advance: vending machine breakfast, vending machine lunch. I'm already thinking about what I'll do—what I'll eat, who I'll call, where I'll drive—once I'm out.

Charlie and I met two years ago at an ultramarathon in Tennessee, several months before Charlie was convicted of mortgage fraud and sentenced to twenty-one months at the Federal Correctional Institution (FCI) Beckley, in Beaver, West Virginia.

Charlie is a cat of many lives: once-upon-a-time crack addict, father of two, professional repairer of hail damage, TV producer, motivational speaker, documentary film star, and—for the past twenty years—one of the strongest ultradistance runners in the world. Charlie started running in eighth grade: *I was awkward and gangly and self-conscious pretty much all the time, except when I was running,* he wrote to me once. *Running made me feel free and smooth and happy.*

Charlie's accomplishments are well known in the ultrarunning community: he's run across Death Valley; he's run across the Gobi; he's run across America. He has trekked hundreds of miles through the jungles of Borneo and even more through the Amazon. He's climbed Mount McKinley. In 2006 and 2007, he ran forty-six hundred miles across the Sahara. The journey was documented in a film and it was this film, incidentally, that set his legal nightmare in motion.

The story of Charlie's arrest and conviction is long and harrowing, but here are the basics: an IRS agent named Robert Nordlander started wondering about Charlie's finances after watching the Sahara film. He wanted to know: how does a guy like that support all his adventures? I've tried to understand Nordlander's curiosity as vocational instinct. Perhaps he wonders how strangers pay their taxes the same way I wonder how strangers get along with their mothers, or what secrets they keep from their spouses.

Nordlander opened an investigation, and he didn't find anything wrong with Charlie's taxes. But instead of closing the case, he pushed further. He authorized garbage dives. He authorized tactics that wouldn't have been possible before the Patriot Act. He started looking into Charlie's properties. He sent a female undercover agent—rigged with wires—to ask Charlie out to lunch. Charlie was single at the time. He said yes. He tried to impress. He said his broker had filled out a few "liar loans"—standard shorthand for stated-income loans—and that non-confession pretty much sealed the deal. In October 2010, Charlie was convicted of twelve counts of mail, bank, and wire fraud. Nordlander had won his case at last.

Charlie's case was also part of a much larger story: the fallout of the American subprime mortgage crisis. His conviction, one imagines, was largely fueled by the general knowledge that things had gone terribly wrong and the sense that people should be held accountable. So Charlie was held accountable. He was held accountable for something millions of people did, something he still alleges—

with compelling evidence—he didn't do. He became a convenient scapegoat for the inevitable collapse of a system fueled by recklessness and greed.

At the time of his arraignment, Charlie was engaged. His engagement didn't survive the trial. He was imprisoned a state away from his teenage sons in North Carolina. He lost his corporate sponsorships. He lost two years of racing. He lost the right of motion. He lost—as he'd tell me later, quite simply—a lot.

I first wrote Charlie a letter because I was fascinated by his life. It gave me a sense of vertigo to know that when we'd met, in the hills of Tennessee, he'd had no idea what was about to happen, how everything was going to change. I wondered what incarceration was like for him. *Running made me feel free and smooth and happy.* His body was a body that found solace in moving itself across territory—across deserts and jungles and entire nations. The core of his life pointed its finger at the very fact of what incarceration *does*, which is to keep someone in one place. I wanted to know: What happens when you confine a man whose whole life is motion?

One thing that happens is you turn him into a good pen pal. Over the course of our correspondence, Charlie was smart and funny and honest. He steered himself away from anger about his incarceration, but he did so with such intentionality, such earnest and visible effort, that the anger itself emerged as a negative shape carved in the margins. Charlie described it as a cliff; he had to pull himself back from the brink. *My anger is immense and I hate the feeling that I am losing control, which happens mostly when I let that anger breathe.* He looked for what he could salvage: *Like all difficult things, if we can remain open . . . something positive will come. That said, I am still a bit baffled about what good will come from this for me. I lost a lot.*

He wrote about his mother, who was slipping into dementia: *I miss her. I can say that it's unfair for me to be away from her and it would be true.* He wrote about women: *I have never gone this long in my adult life without sex. I don't think I could have ever gone a year alone out there.*

"Out there," incidentally, was a phrase I heard frequently at the Barkley Marathons, the ultrarun where I first met Charlie. It's a brutal race of around 125 miles (it changes year-to-year) through the briar-studded hills of Tennessee. At Barkley, "out there" meant in the wilderness, on the course, getting lost or getting found or whacking your way through underbrush. "Out there" meant you were in motion, doing the thing, winning or getting beaten. "In here," in prison, was the opposite of all that; it was never getting lost, never going where you hadn't already been.

Some weeks Charlie's letters were written from a low-down place: *My mother is getting worse, my knee is getting worse, my attitude is getting worse.* Or: *Today I awoke full of fear.*

He was forced to stop running on the prison track because of an injury that turned into a Baker's cyst, a huge swelling behind his knee. He wrote about the incredible frustration of trying to get treatment: *I have spent more than 90 days just trying to see the doctor. The neglect here is almost unimaginable.*

At Christmas, he sent a photocopied cartoon: a bearded Santa behind bars staring at a puny tree. "Wish You Were Here" was crossed out and replaced by "Wish I Was There."

Writing to Charlie often made me feel guilty. I wrote about something as simple as walking around my neighborhood, with its methadone clinic and its blossoming pear trees, and felt like there was no way to communicate my world to Charlie that wasn't rubbing salt into the central wound of his life. I wrote about running in the rain—*by the end I was so soaked I didn't even feel separate from it*—and how running in New Haven rain reminded me of running in Virginia rain with my brother, past a fish factory on the Chesapeake, after our grandfather died. *Maybe I'm an asshole to write to you about running,* I wrote, but sent the letter anyway. I thought it might connect to something Charlie had mentioned about running around the prison's gravel track during a storm. It was the best time to run, he'd written, because everyone else went inside. It was the only time he got to be alone. Talking on the phone with Charlie was even stranger: a voice announced, at even intervals, *You are talking to an inmate at a Federal Correctional Facility,* and I walked down Trumbull Street in the twilight while he sat somewhere—in a little plastic booth? I couldn't even picture it— and when we got off the phone, I ate roasted trout at the nicest restaurant in town while he headed off for another stretch of top-bunk reading into the late night.

I liked when we wrote about the past, because it meant we were on equal footing—or rather, he had more past than I did. As he put it, more life experience under his singlet. We both wrote about drinking and using, and stopping drinking and using. Charlie wrote about being an addict with twenty years of sobriety in a prison where he suspected no one else—out of more than four hundred men—had gotten clean before arriving. In his twenties, Charlie ran a hail-repair business that took him all over the country—chasing nasty weather and its comet trail of damage, chasing eight balls in the worst neighborhoods of shitty midwestern cities. He hit bottom getting shot at by angry dealers in the wrong part of Wichita. He would have gotten more time for what he was guilty of back then than he got for what he's innocent of now.

I wrote about the one-legged traveling magician I'd met in Nicaragua, years before, who was a drunk and whose drinking made me unspeakably sad; how I thought of him years later—when I tripped, drunk, on a pair of crutches of my own. I wrote about trying to take a girl, newly sober, out to a raptor refuge near Iowa City—*To see the wounded owls!* I'd promised her, as if these broken birds were some wonder of the world—and how I'd gotten lost, and driven in circles until we finally sat on a bench smoking cigarettes instead, and how I felt like a failure because I wanted to make sobriety seem full of possibility but instead I'd made it seem full of disappointment.

For a week, in the spring, Charlie and I wrote letters every day. We made a ritual out of noticing. We focused on particulars. He described an argument about an unpaid debt, a bigger guy approaching a smaller guy: "Blood on my knife or shit on my dick, I *will* collect what I'm owed." He wrote about the evolution of his

Fridays: draft beers for a quarter in his drinking days, pre-race rest days in his sobriety. In prison they were something else entirely: *Every Friday for 15 months, lunch has been a piece of square fish of unknown origin, along with too-sweet cole slaw and potato chips I won't eat. Friday means very loud inmates late into the night, playing cards or dominoes. Fridays mean there will be another movie shown, a movie I refuse to watch because I never want to even pretend that I am comfortable here.*

Charlie wrote about buying fire balls and instant coffee at the commissary, about the correctional officer at lunch who yelled when inmates couldn't decide quickly enough between cookies and fruit. He described how Beckley felt on Mother's Day: *Mother's Day creates a prison full of zombies, walking around in a daze, hoping the day passes quickly.* Mother's Day reminded those men of how they were failing to be sons. Every holiday was an invocation of "out there," the life none of them were living.

Charlie invited me to come visit. He put me on his visitation list and told me the rules: *You probably shouldn't wear Daisy Dukes or a tube top. Also best not to bring in drugs or alcohol.* A woman once came in a skirt without panties. She was, he wrote, *visiting a very young man with a very long sentence.*

I found more guidelines online: I wasn't allowed to wear camo gear or spandex or green khaki that looked like Beckley khaki, or boots that looked like Beckley boots. If there was too much fog, I might get turned away. Beckley gets strict in the fog. The inmates get counted more often. I pictured this fog—this mythic, West Virginia fog—in vast, billowing ripples, fog so thick a man could ride it to freedom like a wave. Every fog count is an act of protest against unseen possibility; Beckley clutches men close—tallies them up, keeps them contained, seals them off.

I found the commissary sales list online in a grainy PDF. You could get Berry Blue Typhoon Drink Mix, Fresh Catch Mackerel, Hot Beef Bites, a German Chocolate Cookie Ring. You could get Strawberry Shampoo or something called Magic Grow or something else called Lusti Coconut Oil. You could get Mesh shorts or a denture bath. You could get Religious Certified Jalapeño Wheels. You could buy Milk of Magnesia or Acne Treatment or Prayer Oil.

I found rules. There were rules about movement and rules about hygiene and rules about possession. Too many possessions could be a fire hazard. You were allowed five books and one photo album. Hobby craft materials had to be disposed of immediately after use. Finished hobby crafts could *only* be sent to people on your official visitation list. There would be no postal harassment by hobby craft.

I saw what happens if you follow the rules: there wasn't just basic didn't-fuck-up official Good Time (Statutory Good Time) but also Extra Good Time, further divided into Industrial Good Time, Community Corrections Center Good Time, Meritorious Good Time, and Camp Good Time. *Camp Good Time.* Not really.

Heading east on I-68, I feel the highway shift as I cross from Maryland to West Virginia. The land is beautiful, really beautiful—endless lush forests, pristine and unblemished, countless shades of green on hills layered back into drifts of fog. I start thinking maybe coal mining is just a notion someone had about West Virginia; or something they like to talk about on NPR. Maybe it's just a theme for the twisted steel sculpture garden I see to my left—Coal Country Miniature Golf—and not an actual series of scars in the earth. Because this place seems phenomenally *un*scarred, phenomenally pure. Freeway exits promise beautiful, luminous places: *Whisper Mountain, Saltlick Creek, Cranberry Glades.*

I spend the night with Cat, a friend from college, who covers Fayette County for a local paper. Cat lives in a ramshackle house strung with Mexican fiesta flags and skirted by an apron of oddly comforting debris: a pile of old dresses, a bucket of crushed PBR cans, an empty tofu carton with its plastic flap crushed onto the dirt. Cat lives there with her boyfriend, Drew, a veteran of anarchist communal living who now works deconstruction and salvage—taking apart empty homes and selling their flooring to hip bars in

northern states—and with Andrew, a community organizer who
works on land reform.

Their home reveals itself in dream-like pieces: a pile of crusted
dishes, a bone on the floor, a giant spider lurking in a white ceramic
mug, a fabric owl covered in sequins, a square of vegan spanakopita
catching fire in the toaster oven, a dog to whom the bone belongs,
a creek out back and a giant slab of rock for sunning and a garden
too, full of beets and cabbage and spinach-for-vegan-spanakopita
and blossoming sweet peas curling up wire lattice and even the tiny,
barely sprouted beginning of a pecan tree.

I sit with Cat and Drew in a cozy room, under a bare yellow
light and its fluttering density of flies and moths. A tiny flying thing
dies in my spanakopita. I ask Cat what she writes about for her
newspaper. She says one of her first stories was about Boy Scouts.
Leaders in southern West Virginia fought hard for the Boy Scouts
to locate a new retreat center here. They offered to build roads.
They offered tax breaks to local contractors. They were eager for an
industry that wouldn't involve plundering the land.

The Boy Scouts built their retreat on an old strip mine. When
Cat was interviewing the flocks of scouts who came to clear trails,
she asked if they knew how surface mining worked—the blasting
of entire mountaintops, the razing-bare of the earth, the turning
of forest into dirt-brown vistas. The Boy Scouts didn't know. They
were horrified. *But why would you—?* That's when a bigger Boy
Scout arrived. A Boy Scout in charge of other Boy Scouts. He said
the conversation was over.

Cat and Drew tell me how to pronounce Fayetteville—like Fay-
ut-vul—and they also tell me about bigger stuff, like how almost
all of West Virginia's forest has been cleared at some point since
the 1870s—in multiple waves—for the sake of salt and oil and coal
and lumber and gas. But it looks so *green*, I say. I tell them about my
drive south—those lush hills, their lovely curves receding into the
middle distance.

Drew nods. Yep, he says. There's no surface mining near the
highways.

Potemkin Forests! I feel like an idiot. Cat tells me to look out for what they call beauty lines—rows of trees planted along hill crests to mask the vast moonscapes of mine-ravaged land beyond. I am one of the Boy Scouts. I am being told about the wrongness right in front of me. Drew says that some of the land here has been mined so much it's essentially on stilts, barely holding itself up. They call this land honeycombed. West Virginia is like a developing nation in the middle of America. It has so many resources and it has been screwed over again and again: locals used for labor; land used for riches; other people taking the profits.

How can I explain the magic of that house? It was a paradise on damaged land, with its fiesta flags and its flutter of moths, its sequined owl and mounds of embryonic squash rising from whatever earth was left between the stilts—and Drew and Cat so full of goodness, their nerves so awake to this world, explaining it so patiently, inhabiting with utter grace their small fraction of a torn territory.

In their hallway the next morning, I find a different dog from the one I saw the night before. This dog seems friendly too. I don't feel like I've gotten much sleep, but I can remember what I dreamed: I was interviewing a man in a dingy diner and I had just gotten through my chitchat questions and was preparing to get into it— though I wasn't sure what "it" was—when the man rose to pay the bill. I woke with a feeling of panic: I hadn't asked any of the questions that mattered.

It's a dream so obvious I feel betrayed by it. It neither dissolves an extant fear nor illuminates a new one. It simply tells me I'm afraid I'll say stupid things—as I'm always afraid of saying stupid things—that I will ask questions that are beside the point, that my curiosity will prove little more than useless voyeurism, a girl lifting her sunglasses to peer between the bars, stuttering *What's it like in here? What part hurts the most?*

I end up finding quarters in a coffee shop tucked under the gray stone wing of a church. I drive to Beaver. I watch for beauty lines from the highway. I can't pick them out, which I suppose is the point. NPR runs a segment on rural schools in dirt-poor mining counties, while local radio plays advertisements from mines looking to hire.

Mining and incarceration are both looming presences on the West Virginia landscape—both willfully obscured and misrepresented, their growth slopes neatly inverted. Mining is an industry in decline; incarceration is on the rise. The number of inmates in West Virginia has quadrupled since 1990. People with political influence and powerful economic interests allow the state to be exploited by new industries in order to repair the damage old industries have caused.

In the false American imagination, West Virginia is a joke or else it's a charity case; but more than anything it is unseen, an invisible architecture of labor and struggle; and incarceration shares this invisibility, hidden at the center of everything; our slipshod remedy for an abiding fear, danger pinned to human bodies and then slotted into bunk beds you can't see from any highway.

Charlie is one of these bodies. His story is the story of a system that strip-mined the American housing market and peeled away whatever it could, leaving the economy on stilts—land on stilts, subprime-hollowed earth—and balancing an impossible future on dreams and greed. Now we try to live in the aftermath. We punish where it's possible. We take a systemic tragedy and turn it into neatly packaged recompense: time served.

I follow my GPS to 1600 Industrial Park Road. I don't make a right turn into Beckley or a left turn into Beckley. The road simply becomes Beckley. I pass an empty guard's hut and find myself curving between strangely manicured banks of lawn and clusters of forest that remind me of nothing so much as a country club.

I do everything wrong.

First, I go to the wrong prison. FCI Beckley consists of two facilities: a medium security prison and a lower security Satellite Camp. I know Charlie is housed at the Satellite Camp—along with other minimum-security guys, mostly there for drugs or white-collar crimes—but for some reason I think I still have to get processed at the main building. This is not the case. The guard on duty shows his irritation at my ignorance. Before we discover this large mistake, however, he has the opportunity to point out my smaller ones: I'm carrying my purse. We'll need to put that in a locker. I'm wearing a skirt. *He was a very young man with a very long sentence.* I want to tell the guard: "My skirt is long! I'm wearing underwear!" I feel my body as an object and agent of violation. I feel suspected and imagined.

I fill out a visiting form alongside an elderly couple. I notice the woman has a plastic baggie full of quarters and dollars; I feel a kind of kinship. She is also looking ahead to the vending machines—has come prepared to offer her son snacks, at least, and company, if she can offer him nothing else.

I wait while the guard gets off the phone. It seems like he's talking to someone who is about to check himself in. "Self-surrender?" The guard says into the receiver. "You can bring a Bible and your medications." Strange to imagine a man at home, or wherever he's calling from, being told the terms of how he will be systematically stripped of almost every possession, a thousand freedoms.

Once he gets off the phone, the guard resumes telling me things I have messed up: I don't have Charlie's number written on the form, because I don't have it memorized; but he can look up his name, which I have also spelled wrong because I've gotten so flustered, and that's when the guard tells me I need to go back down the road to the Satellite Camp.

At the Satellite Camp, the guards are nicer, but I am still doing things wrong: I park on the wrong side of the lot. I *still* have my purse and I need to put it in my car. I feel like saying: *But up there they had lockers!* I want to show off my knowledge of something. Anything. My purse is a black canvas bag with a yellow dinosaur on it. Officer Jennings is almost ready to make an exception. "A dinosaur exception," I say. Jennings likes this. The guys down here at the Satellite Camp seem open to speaking this way—as humans, joking around. Jennings asks me whether Charlie ever got that cyst drained. I say I'm not sure. I have also failed at being a good pen pal.

I hear them call Charlie's name on the loudspeaker. I'm thinking of the families who've got the routine down cold, who have its every motion committed to muscle memory. There's a certain heartbreak to knowing this minutiae so well: the inmate number, the plastic bag of quarters, the jeans and the hard chairs and the faces of the guards, each one's particular tolerance for humor, the twist and curve of the roads, the eventual selection of BBQ chips or gummy fruit snacks; the motions of greeting and exit, how you might carry yourself differently saying hello and saying good-bye.

Charlie stands at the visiting room entrance: a handsome man nearing fifty with short silvering hair. He's wearing big black boots and an olive uniform, his number printed over his heart. I'm not sure about the rules. Can we hug? Turns out we can. We do. But there are other rules: Charlie isn't allowed to use the vending machines, only I am, so he has to tell me what he wants; and we're not allowed to sit next to each other, only across from each other, for reasons I'd rather not consider. When I look at all the chairs arranged around the room I see there is often one singled-out, apart from the others: the inmate's chair, facing everyone.

Over the course of our visit, my Fay-ut-vul quarters buy us the following: a block of peanut-butter cheddar crackers, a bag of M&M cookies, a bag of Cheez-Its and one of Chex Mix, a Snickers bar, a huge "Texas"-sized cookie as big as a child's face, a Coke, a Diet Coke, and two grape-flavored waters—the second one a mistake, or else a free gift to me from the Bureau of Prisons. Our table turns into a miniature landfill.

It's a Monday, not a weekend, so the visiting room isn't crowded. Nearly everyone stays until three. We're an ecosystem. The family sitting next to the vending machines reminds me to take my leftover twenty cents. Two little girls are obsessed with the thin line of ants near the window, marching easily out of prison. One of the girls starts telling Charlie about a sorcerer, and something about her birthday, a monologue that remains largely unintelligible until she pauses to say, quite clearly: "I hate evil."

Charlie says, "I do too."

When these girls first came in—with their pretty, dark-haired mother—Charlie told me he heard their father got reduced time for telling on an innocent man. *I hate evil.* What do we call a government with marijuana laws so strict that one man has to tell on another so he can get out in time for his daughter's fifth birthday?

The girls seem so comfortable with their father—eager to sit on his lap, laugh at his funny faces, gratuitously court his already-granted attention—but this ease feels deceptive. They must associate this place with long drives, nebulous fear, men in uniforms, and their mother's sadness.

Two frail old white women arrive. One hangs her pink cane on the back of a chair. The cane matches her lipstick. The women are eventually joined by a large black inmate. Charlie watches my face. He smiles, "Not what you were expecting?" He tells me these women are raising the man's kids. They show him photographs. They buy him a bag of pretzels. Caitlin, the little girl who hates evil, tries to grab the pink cane. "Not a toy!" her mother shouts. The old woman doesn't appear to notice. She calmly reaches two orange-dusted fingers into a bag of Cheetos, brings another one to her dry painted lips, and watches her tall friend stare at the changed face of his own child.

Charlie and I spend the first few hours talking about his case. He offers a few theories about Nordlander: probably Nordlander was a kid who got his head flushed down the toilet; maybe he thinks Charlie was the kid who flushed it. I find myself growing restless. Why is that? I feel like I'm in the middle of a story Charlie has already told—which is probably true, but it's also the story behind his confinement. It's the story that shapes everything about his life. Of course he'd want to keep telling it.

I feel a pressure to separate my stance from Charlie's—to make myself author, and him subject—but I also feel it as an act of violence to disagree with him about his own life in any way. I want to talk about his life *here*. I want to talk about who he has become in this place, what it has summoned from him. But I realize my interest betrays the privilege of my freedom: life in here is novelty to me; for Charlie's it's day-in, day-out reality. For me it's interesting. For him it's terrible.

Charlie indulges my curiosity. He tells me he sleeps on a bunk bed in an open room divided into fifty cubicles, like a corporate office, only the partitions are cinderblock and no one can leave. He tells me about the black market currency (stamps) and where the fights usually happen (the TV room and the basketball court). He tells me how life is different across the street, in medium-security, where he's heard footballs full of coke are tossed over the fence and guards get paid to pick them up. *Across the street* guys are owned and rented. Sex acts aren't seen as gay. "Suck a dick here in camp, it's because you want to," Charlie explains. "Across the street it's because you needed the money, or you were forced." He's speaking softer so the old women behind us won't hear.

I can't figure out if hearing all this brings me closer to Charlie or simply illuminates the gulf between us. Am I learning his world or simply perusing its memorable specifics, shopping like a tourist in the commissary? Sometimes Charlie says, "I'm giving you this," before offering an anecdote. His prison life is only mine at his bequest. I'm giving him my attention and he's giving me something else—not the currency of stamps but rather specifics, intimate access—or its texture, at least—granted by way of details.

Charlie is generous with specifics. He tells me that back in July he spent two days running 135 miles around the prison's gravel track. He timed it to coincide with the Badwater Ultramarathon, a race "out there"—through the flat, baked reaches of Death Valley—that Charlie has finished five times. Charlie only stopped running laps for mandatory count, at four o'clock, and then to sleep. These days he organizes a workout group: a guy named Adam, a guy called Butterbean, and the camp's only Jewish man, Dave, who has an incarcerated wife and a six-month-old baby born in prison. Butterbean has lost fifty pounds since he started training with Charlie, Adam more than a hundred.

But Charlie isn't popular with everyone. He tells me some of the white guys don't like that he doesn't like their racism; and a black guy called him a "white cracker motherfucker" after UNC beat Duke last March. The guy was a Duke fan, and Charlie had been gloating. But Charlie is generally tactful. He knows he has to let the older black guys shush the younger black guys when they're playing poker too loud; a middle-aged white guy has no place telling them to be quiet. But he also tells me he's not afraid to get in another guy's face. You have to be an asshole—just a little bit—if you don't want to get pushed around.

Not getting pushed around is a relative concept when the government is telling you where your body can and cannot be.

"I'm easy to ignore in here," says Charlie. He's learned that weekends are especially difficult—people are busy with their own lives and aren't in touch as frequently. He feels it most on Fridays. I remember how he described Fridays in his letter: squares of unknown fish, rowdy dominoes late at night, no race to look forward to the next day. He can't do the smallest, simplest things—send a text, for example, or leave a message on someone's phone, or have a conversation that isn't punctuated by the constant automated announcement of his incarceration. He lives in another world, and speaking to him always involves speaking across the border between that world and the one we call *ours*, the one we call outside, the one we call real.

Charlie tells me about his notion of "inner mobility," something he picked up from Jack London, which basically involves just that— going somewhere else when he's not allowed to go anywhere. For Charlie, inner mobility means reading books, but it also means following his imagination into other places, other scenarios: "I don't treat it like fantasy," he says, "where I always end up naked with the beautiful woman." Instead it's something trickier, less like wish fulfillment and more like making himself vulnerable to circumstance— one of the many subtle liberties this place denies: the freedom to be acted upon by many frames, many scenarios, rather than the single abiding context of incarceration. The principle of inner mobility is double-edged, opportunity and consequence: "I am free to nap when I want, go for a run when I want, fall in love, jump from a building, or eat cake till I puke," he says. "The most important rule of my inner mobility is that I must follow the trail where it leads and sometimes that is not going to end well." This articulation of desire fascinated me—to follow the trail *wherever*, not just someplace good. Incarceration doesn't simply take away the ability to get what you want, it takes away the freedom to screw up—binge on cake or jump from too high or fuck the wrong folks.

Charlie tells me he stopped asking friends to come because it felt too painful to watch them leave. *Wish You Were Here* is just a Band-Aid over *Wish I Was There*. *Wish You Were Here* is never quite enough. When he tells how that moment of departure hurts, we both know we aren't exempt. No matter how much we talk, or what we talk about—no matter how well Charlie describes prison, or how well I listen—our visit will end. Every moment we spend together gestures toward this horizon of departure—like the perspective point in a painting, everything refers to it. Confessing it does nothing to dissolve it.

Three o'clock is just another hour in the day but it is also these things: the difference between me and Charlie, between our clothes and the dinners we'll eat that night, between the number of people we'll touch in the next week, between those liberties the state has deemed appropriate for his body and for mine. Every guy inside has a dream for when he leaves, Charlie says: one guy wants to sell workout videos based on his prison fitness regimen; another guy wants to run an ice cream boat.

Three o'clock is when one of us goes, the other one stays. Three o'clock is the end of the fantasy that his world was open or that I ever entered it. When the truth is we never occupied the same space. A space isn't the same for a person who has chosen to be there and a person who hasn't.

The neglect here is almost unimaginable—and it's not just neglect from the Beckley staff but from the world itself—the world that has carried on with its daily business while keeping all these men invisibly deposited elsewhere, in a slew of the nation's most obscure corners. On the outside, you can think about prison for a moment and then you can think about something else. Inside, it's every moment. It's impossible to ignore.

The fog count comes at three o'clock—on a perfectly clear day—and some of us exercise our right to disappear and others are reminded that they no longer can. One man exercises his right to run 540 times around a gravel track. What happens when you confine a man whose whole life is motion? I guess that, those laps.

Maybe tonight I'll dream those endless acres of moonscape beyond the beauty lines. Maybe I'll meet that stranger again. Maybe he'll come back to the greasy diner. Maybe I'll buy him a Coke, or a cookie the size of his face, and he can stand for every man who's ever had a story and I can stand for everyone who hasn't listened hard enough. *I'm easy to ignore in here.* I'll ask that stranger every single question any person ever asked another person. I'll ask enough questions to dissolve rhetoric and cinderblock partitions; I'll ask him enough questions to make him visible again, so many questions we'll have to stay in the dream of that diner forever.

Fog counts come when the sky goes opaque and movement feels possible, when the boundaries between the free and the quarantined are harder to see—never dissolved, only hidden—and so the tallies arrive with greater urgency: those who have done wrong are tallied, those who haven't are tallied beside them, and all around the perimeter is a border backed by guns—or the threat of extended sentences—and this border runs like a scar across already scarred land. Prison is a wound we keep tucked in those parts of the country that can't afford to turn it away, who need its jobs or revenue, who must endure the quiet violence of its physical presence—its "Don't Pick Up Hitchhikers" warning signs, its barbed fences—the same way a place must endure the removal of its mountaintops and the plundering of its seams: because a powerful rhetoric insists we can only be delivered from our old scars by tolerating new ones.

⁝ PAIN TOURS (II) ⁝

Ex-Votos

Frida Kahlo wore plaster corsets for most of her life because her spine was too weak to support itself. She painted them, naturally, covering them with pasted scraps of fabric and drawings of tigers, monkeys, plumed birds, a blood-red hammer and sickle, streetcars like the one whose handrail rammed through her body when she was eighteen years old. The corsets remain to this day in her famous blue house—their embedded mirrors reflecting back our gazes, their collages bringing the whole world into stricture. In one, an open circle has been carved into the plaster like a skylight near the heart.

Charles Baxter once found what he called "the last appeal" in a scene from Sherwood Anderson, a woman running naked in the rain, begging attention from an old deaf man. "Her body," he writes, "her last semiotic appeal, or vulnerability, or precious secret—it's all of these things, but it will not be reduced to one meaning—carries the burden of her longing, and becomes the record of erasure."

Frida's corsets hardened around unspeakable longing. They still frame an invisible woman, still naked in her want, still calling to deaf men in the rain. I find them beautiful. She would have given anything, perhaps, to have a body that rendered them irrelevant.

Frida Kahlo and Diego Rivera were married on August 21, 1929. She was twenty-two, he was forty-three. She used to call the two of them *"pareja extraña del país del punto y la raya,"* strange couple from the land of dot and line. In her diary, she draws them as Nefertiti and her consort, Akhenaten. Akhenaten has a swollen heart and ribs like claws around his chest. He has testicles that look like a brain, a penis that looks like his lover's dangling breast. Below is

written "Born to them was a boy strange of face." Nefertiti carries
in her arms the baby Frida couldn't have.

We find Diego like a virus through the diary pages. "Diego,
nothing compares to your hands . . . The hollow of your armpits
is my shelter . . . I have stolen you and I leave weeping. I'm just
kidding . . . My Diego: Mirror of the night." Once: "He who sees
the color" and beneath that, of herself, "She who wears the color."
Sometimes just, "DIEGO." Or "Diego, beginning. Diego, builder.
Diego, my father, 'my husband,' my child."

"Today Diego kissed me," she wrote once, then crossed it out.

It was also in August, twenty-four years after her wedding, that
Frida finally lost her leg. Withered by polio, fractured in eleven places
by the streetcar crash, it succumbed to gangrene and was amputated.
She died the next year, as if this loss—after so many others—was
what she finally couldn't bear. She had forgiven her body so many
betrayals, only to watch it taken from her in pieces. She was fitted
with a wooden leg, but her drinking made balance tricky.

Frida loved her doctors. She thanks them over and over again in
her diary: "gracias al Dr. Ramón Parres, gracias al Dr. Glusker, gracias al Dr. Farill, gracias al Dr. Polo . . ." She thanks them for their
integrity, their intelligence, their affection. She associates their science with the color green. Sadness is green as well, also tree leaves,
and the nation of Germany. She has an entire vocabulary of color.
Brown is *mole* and leaves becoming earth. Bright yellow is for the
undergarments of ghosts.

Riding a bus at eighteen, Frida stood next to an artisan carrying
a pouch of gold dust. When the streetcar hit them, his pouch was
broken open by the force of the collision and Frida's body, ruined
on concrete, was covered in what the pouch held. Gold was sunlight
on asphalt. Gold was the gleam of metal through an open wound.
Magenta, on the other hand, was the color of blood. *"El más vivo y
antiguo,"* Frida called it—the most alive, the oldest shade. *He who
sees the colors.* Frida was the one who had to wear them.

Frida kept a collection of ex-votos, paintings offered in thanks
to saints. These small scenes show angels hovering over the infirm

and the saved, their tiny bodies curled in prostrate postures of gratitude or suffering. Cursive captions offer summaries so brief they seem like gags clamped over the full stories ("I was crushed by a horse; the horse was startled by a snake"). Ex-votos are full of Frida's hope, and her stubbornness: hers was a body pulled almost gravitationally toward injury, but her paintings point ceaselessly at grace.

Two facing pages of her diary show a pair of matching goblets, each bearing the face of a woman: full lips, broad nose, fixed eyes curling tears from their corners. One face is angry, purple and red, bruised and bleeding shades, captioned, *no me llores*. Don't cry for me. Don't weep to me. The other face is alabaster pale with blushing stains on its cheeks: *sí, te lloro*. I cry for you. I weep to you. I leave weeping. I'm just kidding.

Don't weep to me. The wounded one will not permit herself. And yet, does.

Servicio Supercompleto

Near the beginning of *Salvador*, Joan Didion's 1983 account of a repressive state in the thick of civil war, Didion goes to the mall. She's looking for the truth of a country held in its aisles, and also tablets to purify her drinking water. She doesn't find the tablets, but she does find everything else: imported foie gras and beach towels printed with maps of Manhattan, cassette tapes of Paraguayan music, vodka bottles packaged with stylish glasses. She writes:

> This was a shopping center that embodied the future for which El Salvador was presumably being saved, and I wrote it down dutifully, this being the kind of "color" I knew how to interpret, the kind of inductive irony, the detail that was supposed to illuminate the story. As I wrote it down I realized that I was no longer much interested in that kind of irony, that this was a story that would not be illuminated by such details, that this was a story that would perhaps not be illuminated at all.

Her intelligence excavates a truth at once uncomfortable and crystalline: In the middle of a war you can't see, you still want to look. You want to squint your keen and cutting eyes at whatever you can find. Because your subject is fear, and fear isn't something with a particular scent or tint, only something in the air that makes it difficult to breathe. It won't respond to any name when you call it into the light.

Every night in El Salvador, people were being picked up in trucks and killed. Their bodies were being thrown in landfills while Didion stood looking at a row of imported vodkas, thinking, *What?* Just pointing at them, because they were there, and what right did they have?

Irony is easier than hopeless silence but braver than flight. The problem is that sometimes your finger shakes as you gesture, there is no point to point to, and maybe you can't point anywhere—or at least not at anything visible.

I have often found myself in the role that Didion casts aside—the aisle-wandering, detail-pillaging self, who comes for water-purifying tablets and leaves with the price-tagged CliffsNotes of a country's suffering. More specifically, reading her, I find myself in a Bolivian supermarket in 2007, taking notes:

Beatles playing dubbed on the loudspeakers: Hola, Jude. An aisle devoted entirely to canned milk. Bella Holandesa with a ruddy Dutch farm girl. Cereals made especially for old people and athletes—ancianos and deportistas—and a box of estrellas de avena, like the Cracklin' Oat Bran I used to eat endlessly in college, except: Stars! Bags of mayonesa as large as infants, twenty-nine hundred cubic centimeters, and a box of Sopa Naranja made of powdered pumpkins and carrots. An entire row of canned salads: Ensaladas de California and Rusa, both full of "aromas naturales." Anything that advertises salsa Americana contains white wine. From the personal ads in Correo del Sur: *Yosselin is thin and discreet. Janeth offers "servicio supercompleto con una señorita superatractiva."*

Two months later the same newspaper, *Correo del Sur,* ran a piece on a group of sex workers on strike in El Alto, the sprawling city of brick shacks on the altiplano above La Paz. The bars and brothels where these women worked had been vandalized. They sat in protest for days outside a local health clinic. *Servicios supercompletos.* They sewed their lips together with thread.

I look back at my notes: canned salad and powdered pumpkins. I have trouble remembering the point. Metonymy shrugs its shoulders. So does metaphor. The white space between details overwhelms whatever significance they were supposed to bear, whatever pleasure they were meant to provide.

We can declare the facts. We can turn away from the beach towels and say: the Salvadorean army killed a thousand people in the village of Mozote. Or, four church workers were raped. Or, the US government gave the army that did these things $1.5 million a day. But these facts are lined on shelves as well, necessarily chosen and arranged, assigned value by explanations neatly stuck where prices might have been.

So we persist. We say, once more: those Bolivian women sewed their lips shut for days. They threaded needles through their skin to stop their speech, to show what good speaking had done them.

A thousand meters below El Alto—in La Paz, during January—the Bolivians hold a traditional festival called Alasitas. For three weeks, markets around the Parque Urbano are full of tiny objects, tiny everything: tiny horses, tiny computers, tiny diplomas, tiny houses, tiny Jeeps, tiny llamas and tiny llama steaks, tiny passports. People buy models of whatever they need most: a new house, a new farm animal, enough food to last the year. They offer their miniature figurines to a miniature man—Ekeko the midget, the Aymara god of abundance, a smoking doll cloaked in bright wool. They pin their miniature desires to his miniature poncho.

We often mistake the shrunken for the cute, but there is nothing cute or quaint about the force of what is requested here, what is given shape. I imagine the contents of Didion's mall arranged like one of these displays, objects pinned to a vast poncho spread across wide shoulders of sky, bright cloth stuccoed with vodka and foie gras.

It would be a panel of material dreams, or dreamed materials—

the future for which El Salvador was presumably being saved—an impossible horizon of luxuries at the end of deprivation. It would be an unbounded map, this spread of yearning, too broad to see in its entirety. Except, the thing is—you *can* see it here, in the Parque Urbano, because it's small. It's just ordinary objects you can hold in the palm of your hand. No irony for miles. These details of desire don't offer illumination so much as insistence—on dream, or delusion, or both: a dwarf god with his freight of tiny prayers, a boundless longing finally visible in full, in scale.

The Broken Heart of James Agee

Many nights that autumn I went to a bar where the floor was covered with peanut shells, and I drank, and I read James Agee. Liquor carried his vision of trauma all through me, twisted me pliable to the loss, and I wasn't afraid to think like this—*pliable to the loss*—because I was drunk, and drunk meant sentiment was not only permissible but imperative. It was boundless.

Turns out *Let Us Now Praise Famous Men* wasn't about famous men. It was about bedbugs and mildewed bridal caps and farmhouses like cracked nipples on the land. It was about how Agee wanted to fuck one of the women he was writing about. Also, it was about guilt. Mainly it was about guilt.

Originally, it was a magazine article gone rogue. In 1936, *Fortune* magazine told Agee to write a journalistic piece about sharecroppers in the Deep South, and he gave them a spiritual dark night of the soul instead. They rejected it. He wrote another four hundred pages.

It's a hard book to classify: it's got sections that don't seem to belong together: discussions of cotton prices and denim overalls and the soul as an angel nailed to a cross: it uses colons somewhat like this sentence does: rabidly. It's so long-winded and beautiful you want to shake it by the bones of its gorgeous shoulders and make it stop. But the difficulty of closure is one of its obsessions: the endlessness of labor and hunger. It's trying to tell a story that won't end.

I was trying, at the time I read it, to tell a story of my own. I'd recently returned to America after living in Nicaragua, where I'd been robbed and punched in the face one night, drunk. My nose had been broken, then partly fixed by an expensive surgeon in Los Angeles. I'd moved to New Haven, where it seemed like someone was always getting mugged. I was afraid to walk alone in the dark. "Nearly all is cruelly stained," Agee wrote, "in the tensions of physical need." There's a notion we absorb about suffering—that it should expand us, render us porous—but this didn't happen to me. I felt shrunk. Damage became fear. It became an insistence. I read Agee thinking about his own guilt when he was supposed to be thinking about three Alabama families, and I thought about myself when I was supposed to be thinking about Agee.

Or else, I thought of everyone who wasn't me, back on the streets of Granada. I thought of the boys I'd tutored some afternoons—glue addicted and homeless, with their runny noses and loose pants—catching them as they prowled the cantinas of Calle Calzada looking for money and company. I thought of Luis, who'd fallen asleep on the steps of the home where I lived—and how I hadn't invited him inside at night, only woken him up, nudged his shoulder, because he was blocking the door. I inspected this memory for the shown seams of a moral: What should I have done? Maybe Agee kept writing because he was looking for the stitching of a moral, too. Maybe that's why he couldn't stop.

I loved getting sad about Agee because his sadness wasn't mine. My face was claustrophobic and Agee was something else. He was something I wasn't. *Tragedy is second-hand.* Faulkner wrote that. Which meant, to me: families in Alabama hurt more than I ever would, and I could show up at a dingy bar and admit that. This wasn't enough but it was something. Agee felt this about his own book: it wasn't enough but it was something. He writes of a woman's daily work in the cotton fields:

> . . . how is it possible to be made clear enough . . . the many pro-
> cesses of wearying effort which make the shape of each one of
> her living days; how is it to be calculated, the number of times

she has done these things, the number of times she is still to do
them; how conceivably in words is it to be given as it is in actuality,
the accumulated weight of these actions upon her; and what this
cumulation has made of her body; and what it has made of her
mind and of her heart and of her being.

Empathy is contagion. Agee catches it and passes it to us. He
wants his words to stay in us as "deepest and most iron anguish
and guilt." They have stayed; they do stay; they catch as splinters,
still, in the open, supplicating palms of this essay. If it were possible,
Agee claims, he wouldn't have used words at all: "If I could do it, I'd
do no writing at all here." In this way, we are prepared for the four
hundred pages of writing that follow. "A piece of the body torn out
by the roots," he continues, "might be more to the point."

Agee doesn't offer actuality. He only wonders what this actuality might look like—an adequate description, *what this cumulation
has made*—and suspends that possibility in the margins of his book:
everything he can't manage. On the question of poverty and its effect
on consciousness, he is merciless: "the brain is quietly drawn and
quartered." His book does the same to its story, slicing it to pieces
and putting it back together in fragments: the house, the dawn, the
animals, the men, Communism, children. He calls his work "the effort to perceive simply the cruel radiance of what is."

What is, it seems, was broken, so Agee broke his book to fit. Subject
holds structure in its thrall. Poverty pulls apart consciousness—
dissolved into bodily necessity and stricture—and Agee pulls apart
narrative. *Drawn and quartered.* He doesn't think he'll do his subjects
justice: "I feel sure in advance that any efforts, in what follows, along
the lines I have been speaking of, will be failures." He chokes on his
words, interrupted by the commas and clauses of his own apologies.
He stutters here. He stutters often.

I found it hard to talk about getting hurt. I kept trying to make
it something larger than itself, that single moment in the street, to
make it part of a pattern. The easiest pattern was guilt. My hand
had been on a sleeping boy's shoulder, shaking him awake. What

does concrete make you dream? I dream of that boy in circles. I dream of where my hand was. I could think forever about the man who hit me—how little he had, most likely, and how big a difference it might have made to him to sell my little digital camera wherever he sold my little digital camera, that camera I would have given him easily just to keep his hand from striking my face.

Agee went somewhere to look at poverty, and tried to take the damage onto himself, to strip away its metaphors and get to some clean, torn truth beneath—"the literal feeling by which the words a broken heart are no longer poetic, but are merely the most accurate possible description." What was broken in me that fall wasn't poetry. My face wasn't useful as metaphor or aperture. It was only the accurate description of where a hand had been.

It doesn't seem right to say Agee risked sentimentality. Better to say he could smell it from a mile off and clawed his way into it anyway. He thrust it before him like an obscenity, forcing everyone to see how his outrage had driven him to the embarrassment of such hyperbole. I felt infected by it.

What good is guilt? Agee asked. We ask. We like the sound of the question. It puts a crude finger on a heartbeat in us that won't stop racing, a pulse broken in sympathy. It makes us talk. It makes us talk about ourselves. It makes us confess. We want to purge something that even confession won't justify. That sleeping boy. Agee drank when he wrote and I drank when I read him. Agee threw himself at the feet of his subjects and I couldn't even bring myself to walk alone at night, with my bone-broken nose and my vodka-flung and fluttering heart. You get drunk and then you get sentimental, or else you get drunk and get hit. I told myself there was something dense and meaningful in my fear—an earned experience, the residue of contact, a cruel radiance—but truly there was nothing but my arms crossed over my chest, as I walked on empty streets, and no one coming after me in the dark.

✣ LOST BOYS ✣

The first film begins with bicycles salvaged from a muddy creek. We're in the woods. Men stand to their shins in dirty water, moving awkwardly in button-down shirts, speaking in ragged Arkansan accents, saying, "Don't let nobody in here," like boys defending a fort, cordoned by yellow tape, except they aren't boys; there are no boys, which is the point. The boys are dead. They say boys killed them.

The police stand over three bodies so unbelievably pale and thin on the ground, hog-tied by their shoelaces, their ghost skin stuck with green leaves. They look like sleeping changelings. *Changeling* means a child stolen by spirits, or else the demon left in his place. Three boys were killed in May, in 1993, and in their place three demons were found, delivered as sacrifice.

The film's opening shots crackle with the back-and-forth of police radio. The officers don't know what to do with these bodies. The film is gray and bleary; the visual quality seems plucked from that strange purgatory just after waking when you are trying to remind yourself that whatever you dreamed—a death, a guilt, some wreckage—isn't real. That failed hope thickens this gray light.

Gradually, music swells under the voices of the police. You can barely hear the men anymore but you can see the darker lines of water on their pants where they have waded into the creek. Two of the boys were drowned. One bled to death on the banks. The music is Metallica, the early chords of "Welcome Home (Sanitarium)." Its volume rises stubbornly, obscuring the sounds of the investigation. It sounds like a kid turning up the stereo in his bedroom to drown out the sound of his father's voice beyond the door.

The Case

Here's what happened: three boys were killed, three more were
charged, and three films were made, by two men who spent more
than fifteen years following the story.

On May 6, 1993, Steven Branch, Christopher Byers, and Michael
Moore were found in a patch of woods behind a truck stop in an
Arkansas town called West Memphis. Three teenagers—Jessie
Misskelley Jr., Jason Baldwin, and Damien Echols—were brought
into custody and charged on counts of capital murder. The murders were deemed Satanic rituals and Damien was called a Satanist.
He and Jason were known for wearing black, loving heavy metal,
and sketching wizards. Their hair was long. They hated where they
came from. They were teenagers, basically, charged with a brutal
crime on largely circumstantial evidence. Two New York filmmakers,
Joe Berlinger and Bruce Sinofsky, decided to make a film—and then
a sequel, and then a third—to show the world how this trio—soon
known as the West Memphis Three—got to prison and stayed there.
The trilogy, called *Paradise Lost*, follows the accused through their
original trials, their appeals, and the years of their incarceration.

The third film was already in postproduction by the time something unexpected happened: the men filed something called an
Alford plea on August 19, 2011, and were released. This was basically the state admitting it was wrong without admitting it was
wrong. The release appears as an epilogue to the last film—and,
though it emerges from an exhaustive legal tangle the film makes
comprehensible, it still feels like an unaccountable miracle: an ending that might have been called unbelievable, had the films been
anything but documentary.

The Place

You see a lot of highways in *Paradise Lost*. You see a lot of highways
because West Memphis has a lot of highways. The town sits where
two of the country's biggest interstates—I-55 and I-40—intersect at

the Mississippi River. Real Memphis is just across the water. These days average per capita income is just under twenty thousand a year.

The film seems fascinated by the macadam arteries of the city. Its camera keeps swooping along the lines they carve, over concrete lots and beige mall roofs, trailer parks and junked trucks on dirt shoulders. Metallica provides the sound track for all these panoramic shots, lending music to the ugliness of it all, the sameness, the irony of being trapped poor in a land full of highways going everywhere else. These aerial views begin to tell the story underneath this story, which is a story about poverty. It's a story about double-wides in disrepair and chain-smoking and chain-link fences and weeds growing through rusted truck cabs and neighborhoods built around the fact of highways and boys who hang out at convenience stores and break into trailers with their girlfriends and mothers with hair gone crunchy from gel and mothers with pill habits and everybody with crooked teeth. Only the teeth of lawyers and police officers are straight.

This is a story about "white-trash" families kneeling at the graves of their sons. This is a story about people who felt invisible before this tragedy brought them into view. It's a story about boys who can't afford their own suits or their own legal representation. They take whatever the state hands them, and they will continue doing this for years—until a set of films makes it possible for them to do otherwise.

Jessie's stepmom sums it up pretty nicely: "If we had money," she says, "do you think these three boys would've been picked on?"

The Woods

The bodies were found in a patch of forest called Robin Hood Hills, a swath of lush green nestled beside a truck stop. It's right next to the highway but large enough to get lost in. The fallen Eden of the overly developed world skirts the fallen Eden of these woods. Robin Hood Hills should summon a merry band of outlaws, but every time I hear it I think of Peter Pan instead. My mind insists on the fairy tale that best applies. Peter Pan means Neverland, where boys never become men.

Boys is a confusing word when you're trying to tell this story: three boys accused of killing three boys, six characters splitting custody of youth but not of innocence.

"These are not boys that murdered our kids," one victim's father says. "They stopped being boys when they planned this."

The trailers for the film show a three-by-two grid of photos: school portraits of the dead boys forming the top row, mug shots of the accused underneath. The visual insistence on this geometric alignment—on the news, in the papers—stems from the same hunger for answers that eventually prompted the conviction: the compulsion to find a symmetric solution to all this mess. Three victims, three killers. A three-by-two grid is comprehensible as a spreadsheet. People crave some web of correspondence, however evil, something captured and framed by right angles, made right, made orderly—in a still, six stills, finally kept still, finally ordered.

The Accused

Why did Damien and Jason and Jessie get arrested? Jessie confessed, is why, and implicated the other two. Confession can be hard to see around but Jessie's confession looks pretty frail in context. He's brought into the station on nothing and treated like a criminal; he's got an IQ of seventy-two, which puts him at roughly the mental capacity of a six-year-old; he's interrogated for twelve hours straight and only the last forty-one minutes are taped. He gets some important details wrong before he's guided into getting them right. He says the murders happened around noon, when the boys were still in school, until he's corralled into admitting they actually happened at night.

I know false confessions happen all the time. I'm horrified by them, of course, and by the fact that many can't admit, can't *accept*, that they happen, and horrified by the justice system that lets them happen, that forces them to happen—and still, despite all this, it's hard to deny how convincing it is to hear a voice confessing to a crime. I feel compelled against myself, listening to the recording as it's played during Jessie's trial. How could it be anything but the truth? Why would somebody speak words they didn't mean? "Western culture," says literary theorist Peter Brooks, "has made confessional speech a prime mark of authenticity, par excellence the kind of speech in which the individual authenticates his inner truth." An authenticated inner truth: twelve hours, a couple of cops trying to do their jobs.

After his conviction, Jessie is offered a reduced sentence to repeat his confession at Damien and Jason's trial. He refuses. He could have years of his life back, and he says no.

Jessie is tiny. At one point, his defense lawyer refers to him as "little Jessie." *Little Jessie*. Not big enough to be a boy-killer. He's dwarfed by the officers who escort him into court. He's dwarfed by his own suit. Michael Moore's father wonders why taxpayer money has funded suits for the accused. "They're in jail," he says, "they should wear jail clothes." This is the tempting tautology of accusation: guilty until proven innocent. Wear your jail clothes until we decide you deserve something else.

Jessie wears clothes that don't fit. He looks like he's playing dress-up. He looks like the little boy he's forfeited his right to be. He's got ruffled hair and he mumbles and there's still some joy and mischief in his grin, when it comes. In his cell, he keeps Hallmark cards from his family lined on a shelf. He reads their messages in a shaky, effortful voice, sounding out every syllable. He's partway between schoolboy and man; he's propped up a magazine picture of a chick in a bikini.

When Jessie talks to his father on the phone from prison, their conversation is wrenchingly banal ("How are you?" "All right." "All right?" "Yeah, I'm all right"), but it eventually gets around to the subject of a hurt hand. Jessie punched the metal toilet in his cell. He's worried a bone might be broken. His father says, "If you can move it, it ain't broken." There is a deep care evident between them. At moments, Jessie Sr. still laughs. The camera gets close on his laughter, on his unstraight teeth. A father takes pleasure in his son, over a telephone line, despite everything.

In an interview, Jessie is asked what he does at night. "I just cry a lot," he says. "And then I go to sleep."

At the time of his trial, Jason Baldwin looks too young for puberty, much less the death penalty. It's heartbreaking. His hair is light blond like an aura around his head, something from nineteenth-century spirit photos. When I watch him, I feel almost broken at his frailty—his teeth as skewed as his mother's, a gaunt woman whose voice seems to chew on itself—and it's in these moments of aching for Jason, at the climax of my sadness, that I catch myself wondering: What if they actually did it? I get a terrifying flash of them in the woods, doing the things they've been accused of—and I feel a pang of guilt, as if I've betrayed them simply by doubting their innocence for a moment.

But here's the thing: I have no idea. I can look at the evidence, as mediated by a documentary, and feel outraged; I can look at the court's eventual decision to overturn its own decision, practically speaking, and I can feel confirmed in that outrage; I can look at the faces of these boys and feel the strength of truth in what they say; but I can't ever *know*. No one can know, except for them—and the person who did it, if that person is out there. So I feel my heart breaking toward a truth I can't be entirely sure of. It's an odd sort of vertigo: affective conviction thrust against epistemological uncertainty.

During his first film interview in jail, Jason drinks a Mello Yello and eats a Snickers bar. This is somehow the saddest part of the scene—sadder, even, than the things he says—to think of how these treats are nothing, in the face of everything, but still the only things he got to choose all day. Empathy is easier when it comes to concrete particulars. I can't imagine being in prison, but I can imagine choosing a snack. So I'm pulled close to the fact of Jason's candy bar—and, once close to this detail, feel suddenly overwhelmed by the split that renders it irrelevant: the essential divide between his incarceration and my freedom. Jason is free as well now, and I wonder what he eats. I wonder what he missed most.

But on screen, still in jail, all he can do is drink a pee-yellow soda. He says he couldn't kill an animal or a person. He talks about his iguana. It's his favorite of all his pets. I understand the detail of this iguana as an instance of editorial construction: how can you see a boy who looks ten years old, talking about his iguana, and believe he's a murderer? I'm aware that the filmmakers are essentially deploying this moment—how it proclaims Jason's innocence more effectively, affectively, than his own denial—but I'm also complicit in the vision they've offered me. I believe what Jason says about his iguana. I believe what he says about not killing those boys. His lawyer asks him: What does he want to do once the trial is over? Maybe go to Disneyland, he says. He's never been on a trip except to some mineral springs nearby. Sounds like *hero springs* in his mumbling, though he might have just said *hot*. I want to picture Jason Baldwin on a trip. I want to be inside his head when he hears "Not guilty," and I want to follow him on an airplane all the way to Anaheim. This is one of the delusions documentary invites: if it's all edited anyway, if it's all artifact, couldn't it take another turn? Couldn't there be another ending?

On the witness stand, Damien is asked about his name. He gave it to himself. The question he is not asked is "Did you name yourself for the devil?" But the possibility is clearly on the table. It turns out Damien named himself after Father Damien, a Catholic priest who ministered to lepers in Hawaii and eventually died of their disease. It would be nice to find some parallel here—an illumination, at least a segue—but there is no parallel. Defendant Damien hasn't ministered to any lepers. His tragedy doesn't lie in the heroism of his vocation but in its absence—the negative space, those lives unlived, which is to say: the definition of incarceration itself.

Damien could have ministered to anyone, anywhere, but he was kept to one place, one single *here*, where he ministered to no one. Not that his life didn't happen in prison—he speaks beautifully of his meditation practice and his reading, his relationships with other men on death row—but that this life could have happened elsewhere. It haunts his story as a thousand empty margins.

In 2005, Damien self-published a memoir called *Almost Home*. The cover shows a photo of his face, bleached and wide eyed, behind columns of vertical lettering that summon the stark lines of prison bars. The tone is immediate and engaging, sharp with insights and the disquieting heft of specifics, outhouses and clandestine sex. Sentiment rushes, as with Jason's candy bar, toward particulars: the names of pets, the young love for Cyndi Lauper, a stepfather who once punched the family Chihuahua, Pepper, because it jumped onto the bed while he was praying.

The memoir's mood is oddly light and full of humor, but Damien writes with ruthless emotional intelligence. It's often difficult to read. Of the heartbroken mother we see on film, he says: "She knows very little about me, but makes up stories so she can seem closer to me than she truly is. It gains her more attention." Of his girlfriend at the time of his arrest, the mother of his child: "There wasn't much of a courtship and no scenes of seduction . . . I began sleeping with [her] just because she was there." I remember her from the films—red-haired and pretty, angry—dandling her baby distractedly and running from the courtroom during sentencing. Damien knows the story he could tell about this girl—the story, in many ways, we are expecting: innocent passion shadowed by tragedy, young love broken by circumstance. But he refuses the story line loaded with sentiment and tells the one that happened instead.

It feels like a betrayal of the films, in certain ways, to read the memoir—to see Damien's mother exposed as something more human than just a grieving woman, to see the mother of his child exposed as something more than suffering Madonna, to see Damien himself exposed as harsh. It made me realize what I already knew, on some level, about all these guys, or myself in relation to them: because I want them to be innocent, I need them to be saints.

The Parents

Pam Hobbs, mother of Steve Branch, is a pretty and flustered woman who wears floral-print dresses to the trial. She seems unhinged by grief. In an interview with a local newscaster, she wears her son's Cub Scout uniform draped over her head like a turban. She's convinced, at this moment, that the crime was Satanic and the accused are guilty. "Did you look at the freaks?" she says. "They look like punks."

The camera moves directly into footage of boys playing on a jungle gym and spinning on a playground wheel, then pans to a row of empty swings. They twist and creak as if they've just been abandoned, or still hold ghosts.

Michael Moore's parents, Todd and Dana, look like a pair of librarians. They have a daughter named Dawn. Steve Branch once bought her a moonstone. When they are interviewed, Todd Moore speaks to someone just beside the camera. Dana, on the other hand, looks at her husband when she talks. She wants his confirmation in her mourning. Todd wants to know if his son called out for him in the woods.

This was 1993. The Moores are still out there today, somewhere—still cooking dinner and eating it, clearing the table, falling asleep and dreaming. Probably in some of their dreams their son is still alive. They drive to work and drive home and watch comedies and laugh, or don't, and their son—their son is still in second grade.

Steve, Michael, and Chris: each achieved the rank of Wolf in Cub Scouts. Michael wore his uniform even when he wasn't at meetings. Steve had a pet turtle who probably outlived him. Chris was nicknamed Worm because he couldn't hold still.

Requirements for the Wolf Cub badge include doing a crab walk, an elephant walk, and a frog leap; folding an American flag; learning four ways to stop the spread of colds; starting a collection, any collection; making breakfast and then cleaning up; visiting a historic site in the community. I try to guess what landmark these boys might have visited in West Memphis, a place history seems to have excluded from its archives: maybe Eighth Street, known as "Beale Street West" for its Depression-era Blues scene, or the Hernando DeSoto Bridge, a massive piece of infrastructure that helps trucks keep going somewhere else. Most of the infrastructure in West Memphis does this: helps things get somewhere else. Maybe the boys just sat by the highway and watched big rigs roll by.

They'd be twenty-nine this year, a year younger than I am.

Melissa and Mark Byers, Chris's mother and stepfather, are the strangest of the victims' parents. Melissa mainly seems angry. For her, the conversion of grief to rage has been swift and absolute, and the cameras crystallize this alchemy into scripted curse. She wishes the accused all sorts of violence. She says she'd like to eat the skin off Damien's face. "I hate these three," she says. "And. The. Mothers. That. Bore. Them." She taps her fingers like a metronome.

As Jessie is leaving the courtroom one day, Melissa calls out: "Jessie sweetie!" Her falsetto presumably imitates the voice of the man she hopes will rape him. She turns to the camera: "I'm going to mail him a skirt." Her voice sounds venomous but also calculated—not that the anger isn't authentic, but that she has constructed a very particular way of expressing it. She is performing her grief for a set of cameras that won't stop following her around, and her performance can make it hard to believe that an actual grief is dwelling underneath. But it is. Some part of me wants to get angry at her, and I sense that the filmmakers want to grant this anger space. Another part of me remembers: her son died. This is probably the only certain fact for miles.

There's also this: Melissa Byers is most likely a woman who felt invisible and disrespected all her life. The world never cared about anything she had to say. Now, all of a sudden, it does.

On the surface of things, Mark Byers seems like he'd make a perfect documentary subject. He's unabashedly odd, and furious at everything, particularly the devil worshippers who killed his son. He's a tall man with a big belly and a mullet. There's a kind of crookedness to his face, like the residue of paralysis. He says he has a brain tumor. One of his favorite shirts is divided into stars and stripes. His performance of patriotism is striking for the desire it shows in him to come across as good, to be admitted entry into the culture of decency to which he pledges allegiance. (Wolf Scout Achievement number two: *With another person, learn to fold the American flag.*) Byers likes to curse—not just cussing but cursing, full-throated and biblical. He speaks of the fight between angels and demons. He often addresses the accused by their full names: "Damien Echols, Jason Baldwin, Jessie Misskelley, I hope your master the devil does take you soon." He swears he'll perform bodily functions on their graves.

He returns to Robin Hood Hills a few years after the murders in a cowboy hat and overalls, using a machete to hack his way through the tall grasses that have grown where a crime scene used to be. The grass has moved on, the scene suggests, but Byers is in exactly the same place. He's so attached to performing rituals—for an audience, or else for himself—that he's grown impatient to deliver on a promise before its time: *I'll spit on your graves,* when they're not even dead. He makes grass mounds and calls them tombs. He douses them with lighter fluid. "My baby will put his foot across your throat," he announces to the spirits of the accused—who are, by now, the convicted. It's an odd prophecy: *My baby will put his foot . . .* He resurrects his eight-year-old son as a vengeful creature, caught as deeply in this anger as he is.

He lights his cigarette and then drops the match. Flames crackle the dry grass and Byers mashes them with the heels of his cowboy boots. He seems compelled by something powerfully internal and beyond his mastery, but the scene feels weirdly low budget. It's like somebody trying to make a home movie about hell. "You wanted to eat my baby's testicles?" Byers asks the air. "Burn, you sonofabitch. Burn."

By the end of the scene, Byers's theatrics just feel tired. He makes

you cringe too much. He's exhausting to watch. I imagine he got
tired as well. He's furious at everyone: the woman who tutored Jessie
for his GED, the people who say the justice system is corrupt, the
people who say the justice system isn't corrupt. He's furious at an
ever-shifting *they*. His life is lived toward them. They haunt him.
They haunts him.

He has an unnerving way of veering between wounded dis-
orientation and rabid anger. There's a sad slowness to his manner
sometimes, and sometimes a scripted rage, but a sense of abiding
effort, a kind of struggling for purchase, is common between these
modes. He's like a bad actor playing the role of grieving father. This
constant aura of performance is why I think he'd actually make a
difficult subject, even if at first glance he looked like a perfect one.
It seems like he's working so hard to pretend he's something he actually *is:* a father who's lost his son. It's hard to trust any sliver of
raw emotion underneath the stilted emotion he performs—the absurdity of his furious indignation, which robs him of precisely the
sympathy he thinks it will summon.

There's a scene where Byers and Todd Moore crouch in a field
and take turns shooting a pumpkin. For a while Byers steals the
show as usual, calling each boy's name as he kills him: "Oh Jessie!"
"Jason! Blow me a kiss!" There's a stubborn ferocity to the way Byers
invokes the possibility of these boys being raped in prison, as if he's
earned the right to imagine it—to take pleasure, even, in imagining
it. But as with so much of his anger, it feels weirdly stale. He's playing a part. Todd Moore is trying to learn the script. "What kind of
range we got in that courtroom?" he asks, inspecting the gun, like
an apprentice to the craft of Byers's alchemy—his crusade to turn
sorrow to vengeance, to turn three dead boys into six.

I feel betrayed by Moore. I wanted him to be the parent for
whom my sympathy could be complete. Instead it's corrupted
by this terrible sadness at the impulse toward retribution—how
we crave it and how it deforms us, how it whittles everything to
an empty field, a pumpkin riddled with bullets, the crisp *thwick,
thwick, thwick* of each shot.

The Anger

When I watched these films as a teenager, I got drunk. I wanted to feel things without thinking them through. Anger lifted me into a sentimental flurry urgent enough to match what I'd seen. These filmmakers are curators of outrage; they entrust you with an injustice it hurts to hold. So you figure out somewhere to put it. Some folks started a protest movement—*Free the West Memphis Three*—while others gave millions of dollars to their defense. I got drunk and pretended to be a lawyer. I gave impassioned speeches to my hallway mirrors. *This is not justice!* I delivered closing arguments to no one.

Of course, that's not the whole story. Because I knew some part of me was glad for it. For *it?* For the injustice. Some part of me liked feeling spellbound by it. I rose up against it and felt myself shaped by this opposition.

We like who we become in response to injustice: it makes it easy to choose a side. Our capacity to care, to get angry, is called forth like some muscle we weren't entirely aware we had.

Or I guess I should say, *I.* Why project the shame of this rubbernecking onto everyone? I don't want to suggest I wasn't genuinely troubled, hurt, aching for these boys—I thought of them for the next ten years, and wrote Jason several letters in prison, never returned—but I admit that some part of me enjoyed these films. I didn't enjoy what was happening, but I enjoyed who I was while I was watching it. It offered evidence of my own inclination toward empathy.

Back then, when I practiced playing defense lawyer for the boys who were accused, I wasn't thinking as much about the boys who'd died. It was only years later I found their autopsy reports online. All three were found naked, covered with mud and leaves. All three showed "washerwoman" wrinkling of the hands and feet from their submersion in the water.

Their bodies are cataloged in terms of injuries—cuts, bruises, and skull fractures, stripped skin and contusions, "semi-lunar abrasions" above their lips, below their ears, feces around their anuses, the residue of unimaginable fear. The weight of their organs is listed in grams. Christopher's right lung weighed ten grams more than his left; so did Stevie's. The autopsy reports move with chilling understatement between descriptions of the bodies and descriptions of their damage: "The irises were green. The corneae were clear . . . Fly larvae were present in the left periorbital region." The language occasionally turns lyrical. The toxicology report on Christopher includes the following entry on his penis: "Bacterial colonies. A few ghost remnants of red blood cells." *Ghost remnants*. Every beautiful description of violence becomes—in its beauty—a violation of its object.

The word *unremarkable* shows up in odd places. Perhaps, in these documents, it would feel odd anywhere. Stevie Branch's report offers his body in summary: "The chest and abdomen were unremarkable, except for the injuries to be described further below. The penis showed injuries as described below. The upper and lower extremities showed no abnormalities except for the injuries . . . described below." He was sixty-five pounds and blond. His body was unremarkable except for the ways in which it had been brutalized. He was naked save one item: "A cloth friendship bracelet was present around the right wrist."

Why didn't I spend more time thinking about these boys when I first heard the story of their deaths? Maybe because they were past reclamation. So I got angry about the boys who could still be saved.

In a way, I got angry just like the parents of the victims got angry, only the objects of my anger were different. If you're a juror, or a mother, or an ordinary citizen of an ordinary town, you are delivered an outrage—as a witness, or a victim—and you have to purge or off-load it somehow. So you get scared. You fling the hurt wherever it will stick. You make sense of it however you can. The parents wanted three men to go to prison; they wanted them to hurt, to burn, to die. I get angry at their intolerance, their unwillingness to consider any option besides guilt, their insistence on the easiest possible narrative as salve for their pain. The more they insist upon their right to vengeance, the less sympathy I have for them.

In getting mad at them, I suspect I'm doing precisely what I hate the system for doing: looking for a scapegoat. Their faces offer convenient vessels to hold my free-floating notions about a wrongness that cannot be accounted for. Individuals are easier targets than a faceless justice system too large to hate. I remind myself: these parents are only blaming the guys they've been told to blame. Which is another casualty of the justice system—not just robbing three boys of their freedom, but robbing three families of their grief, insisting that they turn this grief to something else. The police and the courts—with their conviction, in both senses, their certainty and their verdict—invited these families to trade grace for vengeance.

With the victims' families, I find myself veering wildly between anger and guilt. I feel such sadness for what their grief must be like—forcing them to live inside such rage on top of their unimaginable loss. They lost their children, and in return were offered the chance to become complicit in a burning.

Prairie burning is the name for what happens when people set fire to the land so that it will grow. It's a controlled devastation, like irradiating cancer cells that rebel against a body, or amputating a foot gone black with gangrene. Years ago witches were torched like fields. Their bodies bore the controlled burn. Their bodies held evil like vessels so that evil would not be understood as something diffused across other bodies, across everyone.

The Trial

It's the imperative of efficiency that got these boys accused and the mechanics of pride that got them convicted. Gary Gitchell, the chief inspector of the West Memphis police, is the face of this efficiency. At a press conference early in the first film, when asked about the strength of his case on a scale of one to ten, he says, "Eleven." He says "eleven" and people clap. They laugh.

It's an eleven the state of Arkansas will overturn, eighteen years later, when it sets these boys free as men. But in the documentary, *eleven* stands, immortalized forever. People laugh at this eleven because they need it so badly. They laugh from relief. They want to

believe in what Gitchell's words imply about the justice system and
the nature of wrongdoing—they need to believe that for every irrefutable tragedy, there's an irrefutable way to make things right again.

"I think the cops just can't find who done it," says Jessie Sr.,
shortly after his son's arrest. He's sitting in a recliner. He has a red
face and dirty hands. He's a mechanic. He looks calm. When Jessie
is released, years later, father and son will bow out of the public
festivities and get some barbecue instead. But Jessie Sr., trapped in
this moment, doesn't know about that barbecue—doesn't know that
it's coming; or how many nights lie between. For eighteen years of
phone calls, his teeth will show when he laughs. The camera already
knows that, and brings you close to his face to show something animal in his laughter—not something brute, but something having
to do with survival. It hurts to be this close to the simple fact of his
mouth, the white of his teeth.

This intimate attention is constant across these films; it thickens
their world and makes them ache. The same bikes dredged up from
the creek are shown after the verdicts, being loaded into a van—
presumably about to get shoved away for good in some dark storage
locker of evidence. Or the camera lingers for an extra moment on
the steel toilet in Jessie's cell—the same one that bruised his fist but
did not break it. *If you can move it, it ain't broken.* If you can breathe
in prison, you are still living. If you show teeth, you are laughing; if
you can laugh, you are surviving.

This finely textured camera work forces empathy to effuse in
all directions, even where it isn't meant to go. You get so close to
everyone, you can feel sorry for anyone. The angles are exacting and
perceptive, catching tremors of pain on parents' faces during trial,
or flash-fissures of doubt from one of Gitchell's officers on the witness stand—a sudden flick of his eyes, a moment of panic at having
goofed up, at revealing a chink in the system—another testimony
that everyone here is nervous, including the police officers who
seem so smug. Everyone is afraid of something.

The films also do a fantastic job of capturing odd moments of
triviality, the disconcertingly casual texture of being sentenced to

die for a crime you didn't commit. Life can't feasibly be lived as dire gravity at every moment. The films get this. Sitting with his lawyers, Damien goes over a low point in his testimony. He was daydreaming, he explains, and only halfway paying attention to the question.

"Maybe they'll only halfway kill you," his lawyer replies.

Damien laughs. The camera zooms in, as if querying: how could he laugh? And then it lingers a moment, as if suggesting, even insisting, since no response could be appropriate, in the sense of expected or adequate, since *appropriate* no longer means anything here—how could he not laugh? Who cares if he does?

As teenagers on camera, Damien and Jason giggle when they remember the night they got arrested. They were just watching TV on the couch. "Pigs busted in," Damien says, and they shake their heads, as if they still can't believe it. They laugh. *Eleven.* People laugh. Part of this whole saga still feels like a movie to Damien and Jason; even when they're on trial it's still a little bit absurd—and, for one saving moment of absurdity, not really happening. They tried to hide in a bedroom and turn off the lights. But the police wouldn't go away. Not for another eighteen years.

The Bond

The friendship between these boys comes across as something deeply felt. At the hearing that sets them free, Jason will submit a plea he doesn't believe in, admitting legal guilt, in order to save Damien's life. (Damien was the only one of the three on death row.) Damien thanks him for this willingness at their press conference. For the first time in nearly twenty years, they hug. It's hard to imagine what this hug would feel like, how intimate or inadequate—touching the body of a man who'd lost his life, just like you'd lost yours, but was still alive, just as you were, and now free. They lean across microphones, awkwardly, to embrace.

Damien closes his memoir with a simple moment: catching sight of Jason in prison. This was 2005. They were both living in the Varner Unit, a prison near Pine Bluff. They went for years without contact until Jason appeared out of the blue one day, on the other side of a glass wall. "He raised his hand and smiled," Damien writes, "then he was gone, like a ghost." It's a sad scene because nothing happens. That's what they have, all they have: a glass wall, a raised hand—one of them ghosted and the other haunted.

When they were boys, Damien and Jason had an entire world to disavow. There were arcade games to play and curfews to break and trailer parks to ditch, and there was music fierce enough to lend every breakage resonance. So much music: Slayer, Metallica, Megadeth. So much volume. In Damien's memoir, the only relationships that appear flawless are his friendship with Jason and their shared love affair with music. They lived for it. They were always two boys crouching in a dark bedroom, waiting to be left alone, itching for sound.

I've often imagined my life with a sound track. Like we all have. I've heard music bloating the stories of my life, lifting commonplace discontent to the pitch of tragic drama. I think of this bloat as Metallica thrums under the vistas of Damien's story: sprawling trailers and blurred big rigs, yellow crime tape flapping in the breeze. Damien was given a sound track, probably the one he'd always heard anyway, but for reasons he'd never imagined—and it couldn't comfort him during the days of his incarceration because he had no access to a stereo in prison. It couldn't hold his emotions, deepen or soothe them—it can only do these things for *us*, now, as we watch a movie about his life. Surging chords of Metallica aren't the sound track of Damien's story so much as the sound track of *our* story of his story, which is to say: the story of our hearts breaking for him.

The Reason

One of the brilliant narrative betrayals of Truman Capote's *In Cold Blood*, the grandfather of all highbrow true crime, is that the criminals at its center, the men who killed an entire family, ultimately emerge with no motive besides money. This feels like a second death:

it makes the deaths feel meaningless by taking away the possibility of any affective frame that could explain them. The murderer at the center of the book, Perry Smith, is described as "capable of dealing, with or without motive, the coldest deathblows." *With or without,* that casual eitherness, is terrifying.

It's easier, somehow, if there's a reason for tragedy—lust or jealousy or hatred or revenge. We can find in these explanations an emotional tenor commensurate with the gravity of the act. There's something we recognize as human, a motive toward which we can direct our rage but can also understand, at some primal level, as an extension of ourselves.

"I see no motive," says a disembodied voice in the first film, while the camera prowls the forest floor—getting close to the ground as if hunting for it, this lost motive, nestled in tangled tree roots or buried in a creek gully long gone dry. The parents need an explanation. So do reporters. So do prosecutors. There's no motive apparent so motives are found. The press says "Satanic orgy." The parents seem convinced of devil worship. Damien calls West Memphis "Second Salem."

"We tell ourselves stories in order to live," Joan Didion wrote, meaning frightened people need motives. Meaning everyone does.

A preacher remembers Damien saying he couldn't be saved. He hadn't taken the Bible into his heart. Damien self-identifies as Wiccan—which he explains on the stand as "basically a close involvement with nature." Hearing him say this, I can't help thinking of the woods. I think of three boys lying hog-tied. I don't hear guilt, but I hear the connective tissue of imagining—how, faced with a tragedy, you want to put the pieces together any way they might fit. I spend a lot of time thinking about what happens in the minds of jurors. Who were they? What were they afraid of? What did a guilty verdict offer them that innocence wouldn't have?

The films demand point-of-view train hopping as an ethical imperative—just when you've gotten deep inside the groove of someone's pain, you are jolted suddenly into the pain of another. This empathy is thrown into relief by the fact that, in the films, empathy is rare. Which is understandable. The parents of these boys suffer deep into particulars. *Washerwoman wrinkling. Fly larvae. Ghost remnants.* How could a mother live with these details? Anger burns them like fuel. A man crushes fire with his cowboy boots.

These grieving parents are cocooned by anger, the only structure in which they find shelter. They don't have much energy left over for compassion. They wear their curses like garments. *And the mothers that bore them.* These mothers are suffering too.

The convicted men are the only ones who summon much compassion. Damien thinks about the three boys who died all the time. "They didn't do anything to deserve what they got," he says. He has a son of his own, born a few months after his arrest.

"I have anger sometimes," says Jason, after years in prison, "but there's no one to direct it toward."

He acknowledges explicitly what others simply enact: the problem of tragedy without a vector, anger without object or container. There's a moment, in the first film, when Jason is asked what he'd say to the families of the victims. He shakes his head silently, bashful—looking, more than anything, like a boy who's been asked which girl he's got a crush on. He says, finally and quietly, "I don't know." This seems like a startling moment of *rightness,* in a world where everyone seems so absurdly sure of what they have to say to everyone. It feels right to confess unknowing amid voices so quick to reach for conclusion, so eager to clutch the stability of accusation and indignation, the talisman of demon or scapegoat. Now here's a boy they say killed a boy, saying, *I don't know.*

Years later, in a sequel, he has something to say. Has *something*— which means, has what? Has the enduring fact of incarceration, too many beatings to count, a broken collarbone.

Now he would tell the families of the victims this: he understands why they hate him. But he's innocent. He'd want to hate someone too, if it had been his little brother who died. But he's innocent. He says it twice.

Why do I like Jason so much? My heart reaches for him in a way it doesn't for the others. For starters, he looks so young, even when he begins—in the second and third films—to go bald. Also, he looks a little like my brother. *If it had been my little brother,* he said. It works like that. Kin is kind, is a kind of muscle memory. Maybe this is why I can't stand to watch his face behind the glass of the patrol car, getting smaller as he's driven away from the verdict. Maybe this is why I can't stand to watch him getting into the backseat, moving so gracefully in his handcuffs, adept from months of practice. It hurts to watch the fluency of a body acclimated to its shackling.

The Epilogue

The third film in the trilogy is subtitled *Purgatory.* It was named before the saving grace of its ending arrived. In its version of purgatory, certain things remain the same. The DA's office is still claiming *eleven.* The boys still claim innocence. But other things have changed: now John Mark Byers thinks they're innocent too. New genetic evidence has him convinced. His truck displays a WM3 sticker on the back window. He sings the same tune of careening indignation, but his lyrics are different: *They're innocent,* he says now. *It's an injustice.* He's older now. It's impossible to forget his cowboy boots on the forest floor, from the second film, stomping out his own grave fires. *You wanted to eat my baby's testicles.* It's impossible to tell whether he's changed his mind despite his persona or because of it, whether his change of heart is a recanting of his former performance or simply the next act. Melissa Byers is dead. Pam Hobbs isn't sure the boys are innocent, but she thinks they might deserve a new trial. We don't see Todd and Dawn Moore. They're done with documentaries.

Sinofsky and Berlinger started making this third film in 2004. For long stretches of time, eight or nine months, they filmed nothing. There was nothing to film. Which was part of what they wanted to show: for these boys, nothing was moving. Jessie got a tattoo of a clock on the top of his bald head. The clock had no hands. Time was standing still. In certain ways, of course, it wasn't. Damien married a woman he'd been corresponding with for years. They had a Buddhist ceremony in prison. Jason told the cameras he was still living his life. "You make the most of the hand you're dealt," he said, something he learned to believe because he couldn't survive believing anything else.

The Epilogue to the Epilogue

One of the first and only men accused of witchcraft in America was John Floyd of Massachusetts. He had seven children and some land in a place called Rumney Marsh. In 1692 he was placed in an underground prison later known as the Salem Witch Dungeon. The accusation went something like this: a girl held a cloth he had touched, and she swooned. Centuries later it went like this: three boys wore black, and people swooned. There was music they liked, and people swooned. There were three children who bled, and people swooned. A monument in Danvers dedicated to those accused of witchcraft reads: "Say you are the child of the devil and you will not hang." The Alford plea that released Damien, Jason, and Jessie essentially meant they pleaded guilty while maintaining their innocence. They officially conceded that the jury had had enough evidence to convict them.

Here's the funny thing about this case: the films didn't simply document the story, they also became part of it. In physics, they call it the observer effect: you can't observe a physical process without affecting it. The films brought the case into the public eye, pissed off many of the folks involved, and earned the convicted men a slew of celebrity supporters who funded their defense for years. This wasn't a story about three poor kids getting a bad break then getting it rectified. This was a story about three poor kids getting a bad break then getting a lot of money then getting it rectified. Without these films, these men never would have gone free. Which means the films eventually documented an ending they helped write.

Jason resisted the Alford plea at first, not wanting to admit—after all these years—to something he hadn't done. He did it to save

Damien's life. *Say you are the devil and you will not hang.* Evil needs
to be confessed to be contained. Confession pins the possibility of
wrongdoing, contours it to the body of a single rusted knife from
the bottom of a trailer park lake, imprisons it inside the circumfer-
ence of a tattoo on a bald scalp—time standing still, evil confined
to a body, three bodies, and these bodies confined to a place. Until
they were set free. These bodies, at least. We are still left with this
human fact, this need to turn sorrow so unequivocally—so insis-
tently, and ruthlessly—to blame.

Our hearts lift at the final film's epilogue, its *deus ex machina, ex
curiam, ex odeum.* God out of the machine, the court, the theater.
We see Damien leave with his wife. We see Jason reunited with his
mother, who looks even gaunter than she did twenty years ago. We
know Jessie will eat some barbecue with his dad and finally get some
hands tattooed on his clock (set to 1:00 p.m., the time he walked out
of the circuit courtroom). We know the other two will party—as
they say, like rockstars—with Eddie Vedder in a Memphis hotel.
These simple facts feel like impossible miracles. We get hungry for
specifics: What does sunlight feel like to these guys? What about
wine? Or hamburgers? The liberty of choosing how to spend the ordinary moments of a day? Will Jason ever get to Disneyland? Will
he ever take his children? Will he ever have children to take? We
can ask: Where did these boys go when they were released from the
Varner Unit of the Arkansas Department of Corrections? We can
ask: Who remains?

GRAND UNIFIED
✇ THEORY OF FEMALE PAIN ✇

The young woman on the bus with a ravaged face and the
intense eyes of some beautiful species of monkey . . . turned
to me and said, "I think I'm getting a sore throat. Can you
feel it?"

—ROBERT HASS, "Images"

We see these wounded women everywhere:

Miss Havisham wears her wedding dress until it burns. *The bride within the bridal dress had withered like the dress.* Belinda's hair gets cut—*the sacred hair dissever[ed] / From the fair head, for ever, and for ever!*—and then ascends to heaven: *thy ravish'd hair / Which adds new glory to the shining sphere!* Anna Karenina's spurned love hurts so much she jumps in front of a train—freedom from one man was just another one, and then he didn't even stick around. *La Traviata's* Violetta regards her own pale face in the mirror: tubercular and lovely, an alabaster ghost with fevered eyes. Mimi is dying in *La Bohème,* and Rodolfo calls her beautiful as the dawn. *You've mistaken the image,* she tells him. *You should have said "beautiful as the sunset."*

Women have gone pale all over *Dracula.* Mina is drained of her blood, then made complicit in the feast: *His right hand gripped her by the back of the neck, forcing her face down on his bosom. Her white nightdress was smeared with blood . . . The attitude of the two had a terrible resemblance to a child forcing a kitten's nose into a saucer of milk.* Maria in the mountains confesses her rape to an American soldier—*things were done to me I fought until I could not see*—then submits herself to his protection. "No one has touched thee, little rabbit," the soldier says. His touch purges every touch that came before it. She is another kitten under male hands. How does it go, again? Freedom from one man is just another one. Maria gets her hair cut, too.

Sylvia Plath's agony delivers her to a private Holocaust: *An engine, an engine / Chuffing me off like a Jew.* And her father's ghost plays train conductor: *Every woman adores a Fascist / The boot in the face, the brute / Brute heart of a brute like you.* Every woman adores a Fascist, or else a guerrilla killer of Fascists, or else a boot in the face from anyone. Blanche DuBois wears a dirty ball gown and depends on the kindness of strangers. *The bride within the dress had withered like the dress.* Men have raped her and gone gay on her and died on her. Her closing stage directions turn her luminescent: "She has a tragic radiance in her red satin robe allowing the sculptural lines of her body." Her body is *allowed.* Meaning: granted permission to exist by tragedy, permitted its soiled portion of radiance.

The pain of women turns them into kittens and rabbits and sunsets and sordid red satin goddesses, pales them and bloodies them and starves them, delivers them to death camps and sends locks of their hair to the stars. Men put them on trains and under them. Violence turns them celestial. Age turns them old. We can't look away. We can't stop imagining new ways for them to hurt.

Susan Sontag has described the heyday of a "nihilistic and sentimental" nineteenth-century logic that found appeal in female suffering: "Sadness made one 'interesting.' It was a mark of refinement, of sensibility, to be sad. That is, to be powerless." This appeal mapped largely onto illness: "Sadness and tuberculosis became synonymous," she writes, and both were coveted. Sadness was interesting and sickness was its handmaiden, providing not only cause but also symptoms and metaphors: a racking cough, a wan pallor, an emaciated body. "The melancholy creature was a superior one: sensitive, creative, a being apart," she writes. Sickness was "a becoming frailty . . . symbolized an appealing vulnerability, a superior sensitivity [and] became more and more the ideal look for women."

I was once called a wound dweller. It was a boyfriend who called me that. I didn't like how it sounded. It was a few years ago and I'm still not over it. (It was a wound; I dwell.) I wrote to a friend:

> I've got this double-edged shame and indignation about my bodily ills and ailments—jaw, punched nose, fast heart, broken foot etc. etc. etc. On the one hand, I'm like, Why does this shit happen to me? And on the other hand, I'm like, Why the fuck am I talking about this so much?

I guess I'm talking about it because it happened. Which is the tricky flip side of Sontag's critique. We may have turned the wounded woman into a kind of goddess, romanticized her illness and idealized her suffering, but that doesn't mean she doesn't happen. Women still have wounds: broken hearts and broken bones and broken lungs. How do we talk about these wounds without glamorizing them? Without corroborating an old mythos that turns female trauma into celestial constellations worthy of worship—*thy ravish'd hair / Which adds new glory to the shining sphere*—and rubbernecks to peer at every lady breakdown? *Lady Breakdown*: a flavor of aristocracy, a gaunt figure lurking lovely in the shadows.

The moment we start talking about wounded women, we risk transforming their suffering from an aspect of the female experience into an element of the female constitution—perhaps its finest, frailest consummation. The old Greek Menander once said: "*Woman is a pain that never goes away.*" He probably just meant women were trouble. But his words work sideways to summon the possibility that being a woman *requires* being in pain; that pain is the unending glue and prerequisite of female consciousness. This is a notion as old as the Bible: *I will greatly increase your pains in child-birthing; with pain you will give birth to children.*

A 2001 study called "The Girl Who Cried Pain" tries to make sense of the fact that men are more likely than women to be given medication when they report pain to their doctors. Women are more likely to be given sedatives. This trend is particularly unfortunate given the evidence that women might actually experience pain

more acutely; theories attribute this asymmetry to hormonal differences between genders, or potentially to the fact that "women more
often experience pain that is part of their normal biological pro-
cesses (e.g., menstruation and childbirth)" and so may become more
sensitive to pain because they have "to sort normal biological pain
out from potentially pathological pain"; men don't have to do this
sorting. Despite these reports that "women are biologically more
sensitive to pain than men, [their] pain reports are taken less seriously than men's." *Less seriously* meaning, more specifically, "they
are more likely to have their pain reports discounted as 'emotional'
or 'psychogenic' and, therefore, 'not real.'"

A friend of mine once dreamed a car crash that left all the broken
pieces of her Pontiac coated in bright orange pollen. *My analyst
pushed and pushed for me to make sense of the image,* she wrote to me,
*and finally, I blurted: My wounds are fertile! And that has become one
of the touchstones and rallying cries of my life.*

What's fertile in a wound? Why dwell in one? Wounds promise authenticity and profundity; beauty and singularity, desirabil-
ity. They summon sympathy. They bleed enough light to write by.
They yield scars full of stories and slights that become rallying
cries. They break upon the fuming fruits of damaged engines and
dust these engines with color.

And yet—beyond and beneath their fruits—they still hurt. The
boons of a wound never get rid of it; they just bloom from it. It's
perilous to think of them as chosen. Perhaps a better phrase to use
is *wound appeal,* which is to say: the ways a wound can seduce, how
it can promise what it rarely gives. As my friend Harriet once told
me: "Pain that gets performed is still pain."

After all I've said, how can I tell you about my scars?
I've got a puckered white blister of tissue on my ankle where a doctor pulled out a maggot. I've got faint lines farther up, at the base of
my leg, where I used to cut myself with a razor. I've got a nose that was
broken by a guy on the street, but you can't tell what he did because

money was paid so you couldn't. Now my nose just has a little seam where it was cut and pulled away from my face then stitched back together again. I have screws in my upper jaw that only dentists ever see in X-rays. The surgeon said metal detectors might start going off for me—he probably said *at* me though I heard *for* me, like the chiming of bells—but they never did, never do. I have a patch of tissue near my aorta that sends electrical signals it shouldn't. I had a terrible broken heart when I was twenty-two years old and I wanted to wear a T-shirt announcing it to everyone. Instead, I got so drunk I fell in the middle of Sixth Avenue and scraped all the skin off my knee. Then you could see it, no T-shirt necessary—see *something*, that bloody bulb under torn jeans, though you couldn't have known what it meant. I have the faint bruise of tire tracks on the arch of my foot from the time it got run over by a car. For a little while I had a scar on my upper arm, a lovely raised purple crescent, and one time a stranger asked me about it. I told him the truth: I'd accidentally knocked into a sheet tray at the bakery where I worked. The sheet tray was hot, I explained. Just out of the oven. The man shook his head. He said, "You gotta come up with a better story than that."

Wound #1

My friend Molly always wanted scars:

> I was obsessed with Jem & the Holograms' rival band the Misfits when I was five, and wanted to have a cool scar like the Misfits, which I guess was just makeup, but my mom caught me looking in the bathroom mirror . . . trying to cut my face with a sharp stick to get a cool diagonal wound on my face . . .

Eventually she got them:

> I have two mouth scars from my bro's Labrador (Stonewall Jackson, or Stoney for short) who bit me six years apart, first when I was six and he was a puppy, and then more seriously

when I was twelve. I needed stitches both times, first two and then twenty-something . . . I was very much aware that I was no longer ever going to be a beautiful girl in the traditional sense, that there was some real violence marking its territory on my face now, and I was going to have to somehow start high school by adapting my personality to fit this new girl with a prominent scar twisting up from her mouth.

She wrote a poem about that dog: "it was like he could smell the blood / in my mouth. Neither of us / could help it." As if the violence was her destiny and also something ultimately shared, nothing that could be helped, the twisting of intimacy into scar. The dog was sensing a wound that was already there—a mouth full of blood—and was drawn to it; his harm released what was already latent. "He has been at my itching," the poem goes, "and cleaned out the rot. Left me / mouthfull of love."

Wound #2

A Google search for the phrase "I hate cutters" yields hundreds of results, most of them from informal chat boards: *I'm like wtf? why do they do it and they say they cant stop im like damm the balde isnt controlling u* . . . There's even a facebook group called "I hate cutters": *this is for people who hate those emo kids who show off there cuts and thinks it is fun to cut them selves.* Hating cutters crystallizes a broader disdain for pain that is understood as performed rather than legitimately felt. It's usually cutters that are hated (wound dwellers!), rather than simply the act of cutting itself. People are dismissed, not just the verbs of what they've done. Apologists for cutting—*Look beyond the cuts and to the soul, then you can see whom we really are*—actually corroborate this sense of cutting as personality type rather than mere dysfunction. Cutting becomes part of identity, part of the self.

A Google search for the phrase "Stop hating on cutters" yields only one result, a posting on a message board called Things You Wish

People Would Stop Hating On. *Seriously the least they need is some idiotic troll calling them emo for cutting/burning etc.* "Emo" being code for affect as performance: the sad show. People say cutters are just doing it for the attention, but why does "just" apply? A cry for attention is positioned as the ultimate crime, clutching or trivial—as if "attention" were inherently a selfish thing to want. But isn't wanting attention one of the most fundamental traits of being human—and isn't granting it one of the most important gifts we can ever give?

There's an online quiz titled "Are you a real cutter or do you cut for fun?" full of statements to be agreed or disagreed with: *I don't know what it really feels like inside when you have problems, I just love to be the center of attention.* Gradations grow finer inside the taboo: some cut from pain, others for show. Hating on cutters—or at least these cutter-performers—tries to draw a boundary between authentic and fabricated pain, as if we weren't all some complicated mix of wounds we can't let go of and wounds we can't help; as if choice itself weren't always some blend of character and agency. How much do we choose to feel anything? The answer, I think, is nothing satisfying—we do, and we don't. But hating on cutters insists desperately upon our capacity for choice. People want to believe in self-improvement—it's an American ethos, pulling oneself up by one's bootstraps—and here we have the equivalent of affective downward mobility: cutting as a failure to feel better, as deliberately going on a kind of sympathetic welfare—taking some shortcut to the street cred of pain without actually feeling it.

I used to cut. It embarrasses me to admit now because it feels less like a demonstration of some pain I've suffered and more like an admission that I've wanted to hurt. But I'm also irritated by my own embarrassment. There was nothing false about my cutting. It was what it was, neither horrifying nor productive. I felt like I wanted to cut my skin and my cutting was an expression of that desire. There is no lie in that, only a tautology and a question: what made me want to cut at all? Cutting was query and response at once. I cut because my unhappiness felt nebulous and elusive and I thought it could perhaps hold the shape of a line across my ankle. I cut because

I was curious what it would feel like to cut. I cut because I needed very badly to ratify a shaky sense of self, and embodied unhappiness felt like an architectural plan.

I wish we lived in a world where no one wanted to cut. But I also wish that instead of disdaining cutting or the people who do it—or else shrugging it off, *just youthful angst*—we might direct our attention to the unmet needs beneath its appeal. Cutting is an attempt to speak and an attempt to learn. The ways we court bleeding or psychic pain—hurting ourselves with razors or hunger or sex—are also seductions of knowledge. Blood comes before the scar; hunger before the apple. *I hurt myself to feel* is the cutter's cliché, but it's also true. Bleeding is experiment and demonstration, excavation, interior turned out—and the scar remains as residue, pain turned to proof. I don't think of cutting as romantic or articulate, but I do think it manifests yearning, a desire to testify, and it makes me wonder if we could come to a place where proof wasn't necessary at all.

Wound #3

Recounting a low point in the course of her anorexia, Caroline Knapp describes standing in a kitchen and taking off her shirt, on the pretext of changing outfits, so her mother could see her bones more clearly:

> I wanted her to see how the bones in my chest and shoulders stuck out, and how skeletal my arms were, and I wanted the sight of this to tell her something I couldn't have begun to communicate myself: something about pain . . . an amalgam of buried wishes and unspoken fears.

Whenever I read accounts of the anorexic body as a semiotic system (as Knapp says, "describing in flesh a pain I could not communicate in words") or an aesthetic creation ("the inner life . . . as a sculpture in bone"), I feel a familiar wariness. Not just at the familiarity of these metaphors—bone as hieroglyph, clavicle as cry—but at the way they risk performing the same valorization they claim to refute: ascribing eloquence to the starving body, a kind of lyric grace. I feel like I've heard it before: the author is still nostalgic for the belief that starving could render angst articulate. I used to write lyrically about my own eating disorder in this way, taking recourse in bone-as-language, documenting the gradual dumb show of my emergent parts—knobs and spurs and ribs. A friend calls these "rituals of surveying"; she describes what it feels like to love "seeing veins and tendons becoming visible."

But underneath this wariness—*must we stylize?*—I remember that starvation is pain, beyond and beneath any stylized expression: there is an ache at its root and an obsession attending every moment of its realization. The desire to speak about that obsession can be symptom as much as cure; everything ultimately points back to pain—even and especially these clutches at nostalgia or abstraction.

What I appreciate about Knapp's kitchen bone-show, in the end, is that it doesn't work. Her mom doesn't remark on the skeleton in her camisole. The subject only comes up later, at the dinner table, when Knapp drinks too much wine and tells her parents she has a problem. The soulful silent cry of bones in kitchen sunlight—that elegiac, faintly mythic anorexia—is trumped by Merlot and messy confession.

If substituting body for speech betrays a fraught relationship to pain—hurting yourself but also keeping quiet about the hurt, implying it without saying it—then having it "work" (mother noticing the bones) would somehow corroborate the logic: let your body say it for you. But here it doesn't. We want our wounds to speak for themselves, Knapp seems to be saying, but usually we end up having to speak for them: *Look here.* Each of us must live with a mouth full of request, and full of hurt. How did it go again? *Mouthfull of love.*

Interlude: Outward

Different kinds of pain summon different terms of art: hurt, suffering, ache, trauma, angst, wounds, damage. *Pain* is general and holds the others under its wings; *hurt* connotes something mild and often emotional; *angst* is the most diffuse and the most conducive to dismissal as something nebulous, sourceless, self-indulgent, affected. *Suffering* is epic and serious; *trauma* implies a specific devastating event and often links to *damage*, its residue. While wounds open to the surface, damage happens to the infrastructure—often invisibly, often irreversibly—and damage also carries the implication of lowered value. *Wound* implies *en media res:* the cause of injury is past but the healing isn't done; we are seeing this situation in the present tense of its immediate aftermath. Wounds suggest sex and aperture: a wound marks the threshold between interior and exterior; it marks where a body has been penetrated. Wounds suggest that the skin has been opened—that privacy has been violated in the making of the wound, a rift in the skin, and by the act of peering into it.

Wound #4

In a poem called "The Glass Essay," about the end of a love affair, Anne Carson describes a series of visitations:

> Each morning a vision came to me.
> Gradually I understood that these were naked glimpses of
>   my soul.
>
> I called them Nudes.
> Nude #1. Woman alone on a hill.
> She stands into the wind.
>
> It is a hard wind slanting from the north.
> Long flaps and shreds of flesh rip off the woman's body and lift
> And blow away on the wind, leaving
>
> An exposed column of nerve and blood and muscle
> Calling mutely through lipless mouth.
> It pains me to record this,
>
> I am not a melodramatic person.

This closing motion—*It pains me to record this, / I am not a melo-dramatic person*—performs a simultaneous announcement and dis-avowal of pain: this hurts; I hate saying that. The act of admitting one wound creates another: *It pains me to record this.* And yet, the poet must record, because the wounded self can't express anything audible: *Calling mutely through lipless mouth.*

If a wound is where interior becomes exterior, here is a woman who is almost entirely wound—*an exposed column of nerve and blood and muscle.* Over the course of the poem, she is followed by twelve more wounded visions: a woman in a cage of thorns, a woman pierced by blades of grass, a deck of flesh cards pierced by a silver needle: *The living cards are days of a woman's life.* A woman's flesh can be played like a game of bridge, or drawn like pulled pork from her body in the aftermath of a broken heart. Each Nude is a strange, surprising, devastating tableau of pain. We aren't allowed to rest on any single image; we move itinerant from one to the next.

Carson gives us a fourteenth nude in "Teresa of God." "Teresa lived in a personal black cube. / I saw her hit the wall each way she moved." Teresa dies when her heart is "rent," and her death is a re-sponse to the constant rebellion and anguish of her living: "To her heart God sent answer." The poem doesn't close with her death, however, but with the impossibility of representing it: "Photographs of the event / had to be faked . . . when the lens kept melting." The melting lens means Teresa can't be immortalized into any single frame, any single Nude, any single wounded posture. Instead her suffering demands our imagination—our invention and necessary acknowledgment of "fakery" and fabrication—each time we try to picture how she hurt.

Wound #5

Here's the CliffsNotes version: girl gets her period, girl gets scared, girl gets mocked. Girl's mother never told her she was going to bleed. Girl gets elected prom queen and gets a bucket of pig's blood dumped on her head just when things start looking up. *Girl gets; girl gets; girl gets.* Not that she is granted things but that things keep happening *to* her, until they don't—until she starts doing unto others as they have done, hurting everyone who ever hurt her, moving the world with her mind, conducting its objects like an orchestra.

Stephen King's *Carrie* frames menstruation itself as possible wound: a natural bleeding that Carrie misunderstands as trauma. Carrie crouches in a corner of the locker-room shower while the other girls pelt her with tampons, chanting *Plug it up! Plug it up!* Even the gym teacher reprimands Carrie for being so upset about the simple fact of her period: *Grow up*, she says, *stand up.* The implicit imperative: own this bleeding as inevitable blood. A real woman takes it for granted. Carrie's mother, on the other hand, takes "the curse of blood" as direct evidence of original sin. She slaps Carrie in the head with a tract called *The Sins of Women* while making Carrie repeat: "Eve was weak, Eve was weak, Eve was weak."

I think *Carrie* has something useful to teach us about anorexia. The disease never shows up in its plot, but we see the plausible roots of an anorexic logic—to take the shame of that bleeding and make it disappear, to deny the curse of Eve and the intrinsic vulnerability of wanting—of wanting knowledge, wanting men, wanting anything. Getting your period is one kind of wound; not getting it is another. A friend calls it "the absence of blood where blood should be." Starvation is an act of self-wounding that preempts other wounds, that scrubs away the blood from the shower. But Carrie responds to the shame of fertility by turning it into a weapon. She doesn't get rid of the bleeding; she gets baptized by it. She doesn't wound herself. She wounds everyone else.

The premise of *Carrie* is like porn for female angst: what if you could take how hard it is to be a girl—the cattiness of frenemies, the betrayals of your own body, the terror of a public gaze—and turn all that hardship into a superpower? Carrie's telekinesis reaches the apex of its power at the moment she is drenched in red, the moment she becomes a living wound—as if she's just gotten her period all over herself, in front of everyone, as if she's saying, *fuck you*, saying, *now I know how to handle the blood.*

Wound #6

Rosa Dartle is a shrew with a scar. "An old scar," says David Copperfield, protagonist of her novel. "I should rather call it a seam."

When Rosa was young, the boy she loved—sinister and selfish Steerforth, who didn't love her back—eventually grew so irritated by her that he threw a hammer at her face. It slashed open her mouth. "She has borne the mark ever since," Steerforth admits, but she does not bear it quietly. "She brings everything to the grindstone," he says. "She is all edge."

Rosa literally speaks through an open wound: the scar is closed, but her mouth is almost always open. The scar itself is a piece of language. As David describes it:

> the most susceptible part of her face . . . when she turned pale, that mark altered first . . . lengthening out to its full extent, like a mark in invisible ink brought to the fire . . . now showing the whole extent of the wound inflicted by the hammer, as I had seen it when she was passionate.

I should rather call it a seam: the ugliness holds her together, knits her skin like it was fabric, gives her shape. It speaks the hurt underneath: she was spurned by the first man she loved (spurned by hammer!) and now means nothing more to him than a "mere disfigured piece of furniture . . . having no eyes, no ears, no feelings, no remembrances." *No eyes, no ears, no feelings.* Just a scar. She still has that: "its white track cutting through her lips, quivering and throbbing as she spoke."

Her scar doesn't make her compassionate or sympathetic, however, only bitter and vindictive. It grants her the sensitivity of keen awareness but not of human warmth. When Steerforth spurns another woman, Rosa takes a rapturous, almost sexual pleasure in the fact of this woman's grief. When someone tells Rosa about the woman's plight—"she'd have beaten her head against the marble floor"—we see Rosa "leaning back upon the seat, with a light of exultation in her face, she seemed almost to caress the sounds." Rosa wants a companion in her damage: "I would have this girl whipped to death," she says. She can't summon sympathy for Steerforth's mother, either—another woman he's abandoned. David is shocked: "if you can be so obdurate as not to feel for this afflicted mother—" Rosa cuts him off to say: "Who feels for me?"

Wound #7

Now we have a TV show called *Girls*, about girls who hurt but constantly disclaim their hurting. They fight about rent and boys and betrayal, stolen yogurt and the ways self-pity structures their lives. "You're a big, ugly wound!" one yells. The other yells back: "No, you're the wound!" And so they volley, back and forth: *You're the wound; you're the wound.* They know women like to claim monopolies on woundedness, and they call each other out on it.

These girls aren't wounded so much as post-wounded, and I see their sisters everywhere. They're over it. *I am not a melodramatic person.* God help the woman who is. What I'll call "post-wounded" isn't a shift in deep feeling (we understand these women still hurt) but a shift away from wounded affect—these women are aware that "woundedness" is overdone and overrated. They are wary of melodrama so they stay numb or clever instead. Post-wounded women make jokes about being wounded or get impatient with women who hurt too much. The post-wounded woman conducts herself as if preempting certain accusations: don't cry too loud, don't play victim, don't act the old role all over again. Don't ask for pain meds you don't need; don't give those doctors another reason to doubt the other women on their examination tables. Post-wounded women fuck men who don't love them and then they feel mildly sad about it, or just blasé about it, more than anything they refuse to care about it, refuse to hurt about it—or else they are endlessly self-aware about the posture they have adopted if they allow themselves this hurting.

The post-wounded posture is claustrophobic. It's full of jadedness, aching gone implicit, sarcasm quick-on-the-heels of anything
that might look like self-pity. I see it in female writers and their
female narrators, troves of stories about vaguely dissatisfied women
who no longer fully own their feelings. Pain is everywhere and no-
where. Post-wounded women know that postures of pain play into
limited and outmoded conceptions of womanhood. Their hurt has a
new native language spoken in several dialects: sarcastic, apathetic,
opaque; cool and clever. They guard against those moments when
melodrama or self-pity might split their careful seams of intellect.
I should rather call it a seam. We have sewn ourselves up. We bring
everything to the grindstone.

Wound #8

In a review of Louise Glück's *Collected Poems,* Michael Robbins calls
her "a major poet with a minor range." He specifies this range to
pain: "Every poem is The Passion of Louise Glück, starring the grief
and suffering of Louise Glück. But someone involved in the production knows how to write very well indeed." I could take issue with
Robbins's "every," or the condescension embedded in "starring," but
in the end I'm most interested in his conjunction. "But" implies that
Glück can be a poet who matters only *despite* her fixation on suffering, that this "minor range" is what her intelligence and skill must
constantly overcome.

Robbins frustrates me and speaks for me at once. I find myself
in a bind. I'm tired of female pain and also tired of people who are
tired of it. I know the hurting woman is a cliché but I also know lots
of women still hurt. I don't like the proposition that female wounds
have gotten old; I feel wounded by it.

I felt particularly wounded by the brilliant and powerful female
poet who visibly flinched during a writing workshop at Harvard
when I started reciting Sylvia Plath. She'd asked us each to memo-
rize a poem and I'd chosen "Ariel," which felt like its own thirteenth

line, *black sweet blood mouthfuls,* fierce and surprising and hurting and free.

"Please," this brilliant and powerful woman said, as if herself in pain. "I'm just so tired of Sylvia Plath."

I had this terrible feeling that every woman who knew anything about anything was tired of Sylvia Plath, tired of her blood and bees and the level of narcissistic self-pity required to compare her father to Hitler—but I'd been left behind. I hadn't gotten the highbrow girl-memo: Don't Read the Girls Who Cried Pain. I was still staring at Plath while she stared at her own bleeding skin, skin she'd sliced with a knife: *What a thrill—my thumb instead of an onion.* Sylvia and I were still obsessed with the density of a wound—*thumb stump, pulp of heart*—thrilled and shamed by it.

Wound #9

Listen to this dream:

> The room was small, but it held all the women you could think of and all the men you were ever scared of in your whole life, passing on the street or just imagining, and all the men you loved the most . . . There were knives and girls skinned alive and kept alive, and one woman screaming but trying to laugh it off to another, "Look what they did to my face!"—and there were amputations performed right there, the limbs cut off . . . and all the things that can be done to a person including the pulling and ripping of everything that we didn't even know we love about a person.

Here's how the dream ends: eventually the girls are skinned to the point of interchangeability—"just bloodiness, like animals turned inside out," like Carson's nude—and tossed from the building while onlookers throw paint onto their falling bodies. They turn all the colors of the rainbow. They turn into art.

They turn, specifically, into a book called *How Should a Person*

Be? Its narrator, Sheila, is one of the onlookers and also one of the girls. (She also shares her name with the author, Sheila Heti.) She is in pain but also making fun of how we distort every pain into the worst pain—*the very worst possible pain*—the worst circle of hell. Superlatives are just another way of proving hurt—an abstraction instead of a cut line on the skin. The dream offers a woman who is aware of how girls try to turn pain into a joke. She makes a joke of this tendency. She is standing in front of you—all shivering and bloody, like a freak on a stage—and cranking up the volume on the pain stereo, pushing on your eyeballs with the force of her mind. Raw bodies turn into painted artifacts. The superlative vocabulary of suffering keeps extending its wingspan.

In college, I took a self-defense class with a bunch of other girls. We had to go around in a circle and tell the group our worst fear. These instructions created a weird incentive structure. When you've got a lot of Harvard girls in a circle, everyone wants to say something better than the girl before her. So the first girl said: "Getting raped, I guess," which is what we were all thinking. The next one upped the ante: "Getting raped—and then killed." The third paused to think, then said: "Maybe getting gang-raped?" The fourth had had time to think, had already anticipated the third one's answer. She said, "Getting gang-raped and mutilated."

I can't remember what the rest of us managed to come up with (white slavery? snuff films?) but I remember thinking how odd it was—how we were all sitting there trying to be the best kid in class, the worst rape fantasizer, in this all-girl impersonation of a misogynistic hate-crime brainstorming session. We were giggling. Our giggling—of course—was also about our fear: *One woman screaming and trying to laugh it off to another.*

Whenever I tell that story as an anecdote, I think about the other girls in that circle. I wonder if anything terrible ever happened to any of them. We left that shitty gym to start the rest of our lives, to go forth into the world and meet all the men we were ever going to be scared of, passing on the street or just imagining.

Wound #10

I grew up under the spell of damaged sirens: Tori Amos and Ani DiFranco, Björk, Kate Bush, Mazzy Star. They sang about all the ways a woman could hurt: *I'm a fountain of blood in the shape of a girl. When they're out for blood I always give. We are made to bleed and scab and heal and bleed again and turn every scar into a joke. Boy you best pray that I bleed real soon. Bluffing your way into my mouth, behind my teeth, reaching for my scars. Did I ever tell you how I stopped eating, when you stopped calling? You're only popular with anorexia. Sometimes you're nothing but meat, girl. I've come home. I'm so cold.*

I called my favorites by their first names: Tori and Ani. Tori sang "blood roses" over and over again, and I had no idea what this phrase meant except that pain and beauty were somehow connected. Every once in a while her songs posed questions: *Why did she crawl down in the deep ravine? Why do we crucify ourselves?* The songs themselves were answers. She crawled into the deep ravine so we'd wonder why she crawled into the deep ravine. We crucify ourselves so we can sing about it.

Kate Bush's "Experiment IV" describes a secret military plan to design "a sound that could kill someone." *From the painful cries of mothers to the terrifying screams we recorded it and put it into our machine.* The song would be lethal, but also a lullaby: *It could feel like falling in love / It could feel so bad / But it could feel so good / It could put you to sleep.* Of course the song played just like the song it described. Listening felt so bad and so good. It felt like falling in love. I'd never fallen in love. I was a voyeur and a vandal—flexing the hurt muscles in my heart by imagining myself into aches I'd never felt.

I invented terrible daydreams to saddle those songs with the gravity of melodrama: someone I loved died; I was summoned to a car accident deathbed; I had a famous boyfriend and he cheated on me and I had to raise our child—better yet, our many children—on my own. Those songs gave me scars to try on like costumes. I wanted to be sung to sleep by them; I wanted to be killed and resurrected.

More than anything, I wanted to be killed by Ani's "Swan Dive": *I'm gonna do my best swan dive / in the shark-infested waters / I'm gonna pull out my tampon / and start splashing around.* If being a woman is all about bleeding, then she'll bleed. She'll get hurt. Carrie knew how it was done; she never plugged it up. She splashed around. *I don't care if they eat me alive,* Ani sings, *I've got better things to do than survive.* Better things like: martyrdom, having the last laugh, choosing the end, singing a song about blood.

I was listening to "Swan Dive" years before I got my period, but I was already ready to jump. I was ready to weaponize my menarche. I was waiting for the day when I could throw my womanhood to the sharks because I finally had some womanhood to call my own. I couldn't wait to be inducted into the ranks of this female frustration—the period as albatross, lunar burden, exit ticket from Eden, keys to the authenticity kingdom. Bleeding among the sharks meant being eligible for men, which meant being eligible for hope, loss, degradation, objectification, desire and being desired—a whole world of ways to get broken.

Years later I worked at a bakery where my boss liked putting on a play list she called our "Wounded Mix." We hummed along with Sade and Phil Collins. We mixed red velvet batter the color of cartoon hearts. My boss said that when she listened to these songs, she imagined being abandoned by some cruel lover on the shoulder of a dusty highway—"with just my backpack and my sunglasses," she told me, "and my big hair."

I started hunting for more ladies singing about wounds. I asked my boyfriend for suggestions. He texted instructions: Google *"you cut me open and I keep bleeding."* Best bathos on the air. I found Leona Lewis: *You cut me open and I / Keep bleeding, keep, keep bleeding love / I keep bleeding, I keep, keep bleeding love / Keep bleeding, keep, keep bleeding love.* Each chorus returns, at its close, to the main gist: "You cut me open." The lyrics could be lamenting love or affirming it; trusting the possibility of falling for someone in the aftermath of hurt, or else suggesting that love dwells in the hurting itself—that sentiment clots and coagulates in bled blood, another version of the

cutter's logic: *I bleed to feel.* Bleeding is the proof and home of passion, its residence and protectorate. This kind of bloody heartbreak
isn't feeling gone wrong, it's feeling gone right—emotion distilled to
its purest, most magnificent form. *Best bathos on the air.* Well, yes, it is.
Turn every scar into a joke. We already did.

But what if some of us want to take our scars seriously? Maybe
some of us haven't gotten the memo—haven't gotten the text message
from our boyfriends—about what counts as bathos. One man's joke is
another girl's diary entry. One woman's heartbreak is another woman's essay. Maybe this bleeding ad nauseam is mass produced and
sounds ridiculous—*Plug it up! Plug it up!*—but maybe its business isn't
done. *Woman is a pain that never goes away.* Keep cutting me open;
I'll keep bleeding it out. Saving Leona Lewis means insisting that we
never have the right to dismiss the trite or poorly worded or plainly
ridiculous, the overused or overstated or strategically performed.

In the reader's group guide to my first novel, I confessed: "I often
felt like a DJ mixing various lyrics of female teenage angst." I got
so sick of synopsizing the plot, whenever people asked what it was
about, I started saying simply: *women and their feelings.* When I
called myself a DJ mixing angst, it was a preemptive strike. I felt like
I had to defend myself against some hypothetical accusation that
would be lobbed against my book by the world at large. I was trying
to agree with Ani: We shouldn't have to turn every scar into a joke.
We shouldn't have to be witty or backtrack or second-guess ourselves
when we say, *this shit hurt.* We shouldn't have to disclaim—*I know, I
know, pain is old, other girls hurt*—in order to defend ourselves from
the old litany of charges: performative, pitiful, self-pitying, pity
hoarding, pity mongering. The pain is what you make of it. You have
to find something in it that yields. I understood my guiding imperative as: keep bleeding, but find some love in the blood.

Wound #11

Once I wrote a story from that open wound Yeats calls "the rag and
bone shop of the heart." In this particular case, my rag and bone

shop had been looted by a poet. He and I had a few glorious autumn months in Iowa—there were cold beers on an old bridge, wine in a graveyard, poems left on pillows—and I thought I was in love with him, and maybe would marry him, and then suddenly we were done. He was done. I knew this wasn't an unusual occurrence in the world, but it hadn't ever happened to me. I kept trying to figure it out. A few nights before the end, feeling him pull away, I'd talked with him for a long time about the eating disorder I'd had when I was younger. I honestly can't remember why I did this—whether I wanted to feel close to him, wanted him to demonstrate his care by sympathizing, whether I just wanted to will myself into trusting him by saying something that seemed to imply that I already did.

After he was gone, I decided maybe this conversation had something to do with why he'd left. Perhaps he'd been repulsed—not necessarily by the eating disorder itself but by my naked attempt to secure his attention by narrating it. I was desperate for a *why*—at first, because I wanted to understand our breakup, and eventually because I realized any story I wrote about us would feel flimsy if our breakup had no motivating catalyst. Pain without a cause is pain we can't trust. We assume it's been chosen or fabricated.

I was afraid to write a story about us because heartbreak seemed like a story that had already been told too many times, and my version of heartbreak felt horribly banal: getting blackout drunk and sharing my feelings in fleeting pockets of lucidity, sleeping with guys and crying in their bathrooms afterward. Falling on Sixth Avenue in the middle of the night and then showing my scarred knee to anyone who'd look. I made people tell me I was more attractive than my ex. I made people tell me he was an asshole, even though he wasn't.

This kind of thing, I told myself, wasn't what I'd come to the Iowa Writers' Workshop to write about. Maybe sadness could be "interesting" but not when it looked like this. The female narrator I'd be depicting in my story—a woman consumed by self-pity, drowning her sorrows in drink, engaged in reckless sexual self-destruction, obsessed with the man who'd left her—didn't seem like a particularly appealing or empowered sort of woman to think about or be. And yet, she was me.

Maybe drunken heartbreak was the lamest thing I could possibly write about, but this was precisely why I wanted to write about it. I wanted to write against my own feelings of shame at my premise—its banality and waft of self-pity, the way in which its very structure suggested a protagonist defined almost exclusively in terms of her harmful relationships to men. The story wouldn't just *seem* to be about letting men usurp a woman's identity, it would in fact *be* about this. My own squeamishness goaded me forward: perhaps self-destruction in the aftermath of heartbreak was a trite pain, but it was *my* trite pain, and I wanted to find a language for it. I wanted to write a story so good that my hypothetical future readers would acknowledge as profound a kind of female sadness they'd otherwise dismiss as performative, overplayed, or self-indulgent. There were also practical concerns. I had a deadline for workshop. Seeing as how the breakup was all I thought about, I didn't see how I could write a story about anything else.

I wrote the ending first. It was an assertion: *I had a heart. It remained.* I liked it because it felt true and optimistic (my heart's still here!) but also sad (my still-here heart hurts constantly!). I put the eating disorder conversation into the story so that readers could point to it—if they needed to point to something—and say, *Oh, maybe that's why he got out.* I also meant the eating disorder to clarify that my protagonist's impulse toward self-destruction wasn't caused so much as activated by the breakup, which had resurrected the corpse of an older pain: an abiding sense of inadequacy that could attach itself to the body, or a man, an impulse that—like a heat-seeking missile—always sniffed out ways it could hurt even more.

I realized that this causeless pain—inexplicable and seemingly intractable—was my true subject. It was frustrating. It couldn't be pinned to any trauma; no one could be blamed for it. Because this nebulous sadness seemed to attach to female anxieties (anorexia and cutting and obsession with male attention), I began to understand it as inherently feminine, and because it was so unjustified by circumstance, it began to feel inherently shameful. Each of its self-destructive manifestations felt half-chosen, half-cursed.

In this sense, I was aware that the breakup was giving me a hook upon which I could hang a disquiet much more amoebic—and not so easily parsed. Part of me knew my story had imposed a causal logic on the breakup that hadn't been there. My ex had been pulling away before I'd ever confessed anything to him. But I recognized a certain tendency in myself—a desire to compel men by describing things that had been hard for me—and wanted to punish this tendency. Punishment involved imagining the ways my confessions might repulse the men they were supposed to beckon closer. When I punished myself with this causality, I also restored the comforting framework of emotional order—*because I did this, this happened; because this happened, I hurt.*

In the meantime, I was nervous about workshop. Would I be lauded as a genius? Quietly understood as pathetic? I chose my outfit carefully. I still remember one of the first comments. "Does this character have a job?" one guy asked, sounding annoyed, and said she might have been a little easier to sympathize with if she did.

Interlude: Outward

As it happened, that story was the first one I ever published. Sometimes I get notes about it from strangers. One woman in Arizona even got part of it tattooed on her back. Men say it helps them sympathize more with certain female tendencies. These men write to me about their relationships: women who once seemed like reckless bitches, they say, start to seem like something else. A frat guy wrote to say that now he "got" girls better. I trusted he meant: understood. Another guy said: *I have always been curious of the psychology of women who tend toward a want to be dominated.*

A Hawaiian real estate agent wrote about his little sister. He'd never been compassionate about her painful relationships with men. *I'm sure that your goal was not to educate men on the psychological nuances of women,* he said, but he felt he could relate to his sister's self-destructive tendencies better after reading the story—*a little wisp of understanding,* he said. I was thrilled. My pain had flown beyond the confines of its bone shop. Now it had a summer home in the Pacific.

I wouldn't say writing that story helped me get over my breakup any faster; it probably did just the opposite. I ended up consigning that ex into the realm of legend—a sort of mythic prop around which I'd constructed this suffering version of myself. But the story helped me weave the breakup into my sense of self in a way that ultimately felt outward, directed toward the lives and pain of others.

And yet—do I still wonder if my ex ever read that story? Of course I do.

Wound #12

The summer after my freshman year of college, my mouth was wired shut for two months while my jaw healed from an operation. The joint hinge had been damaged in an accident—I'd fallen off a vine in Costa Rica, twenty feet to cloud forest floor—and certain bones had been drilled into new shapes and then screwed back together again. The wires held everything in place. I couldn't talk or eat. I squirted geriatric energy drinks into the small opening between my teeth and the back of my mouth. I wrote notes on little yellow pads. I read a lot. Already, then, I thought of documenting my experience for posterity. And I already had the title of my memoir in mind: *Autobiography of a Face.*

That's how I discovered Lucy Grealy. Her memoir, *Autobiography of a Face,* is the story of her childhood cancer and enduring facial disfigurement. I read it in an afternoon and then I read it all over again. Its central drama, for me, wasn't Grealy's recovery from illness; it was the story of her attempt to forge an identity that wasn't entirely defined by the wound of her face. At first she couldn't see her face as anything but a locus of damage to which everything else referred:

This singularity of meaning—I was my face, I was ugliness—
though sometimes unbearable, also . . . became the launching
pad from which to lift off . . . Everything led to it, everything
receded from it—my face as personal vanishing point.

These are the dangers of a wound: that the self will be subsumed
by it ("personal vanishing point") or unable to see outside its gravity ("everything led to it"). The wound can sculpt selfhood in a way
that limits identity rather than expanding it—that obstructs vision
(of other people's suffering, say) rather than sharpening empathic
acuity. Carrie doesn't do anyone any favors. Rosa Dartle is all edge.

Grealy had been craving the identity-locus of damage even before it happened to her; and was happy, as a little girl, when trauma
first arrived: "I was excited by the idea that something really was
wrong with me"—like Molly with a razor at her cheek, trying to
make herself a Misfit. Years later, Grealy still took a certain comfort in her surgeries. These were the times when she was cared for
most directly, and when her pain was given a structure beyond the
nebulous petty torture of feeling ugly to the world. "It wasn't without a certain amount of shame that I took this kind of emotional
comfort from surgery," she writes. "Did it mean I liked having op-
erations and thus that I deserved them?"

In Grealy's shame I see the residue of certain cultural imperatives: to be stoic, to have a relationship to pain defined by the single
note of resistance. These imperatives make it shameful to feel any
attachment to pain or any sensitivity to its offerings. What I love
about Grealy is that she's not afraid to be honest about every part
of her pain: how she takes some comfort in her surgeries and feels
discomfort at this comfort; how she tries to feel better about her
face—over and over again—and just can't. She can't make ugliness
productive. She can't make the wound fertile. She can only take solace in how much it hurts, and in how this hurting elicits the care of
others. In this confession, of course, the wound *does* become fertile.
It yields honesty. Her book is beautiful.

As a little girl, Grealy learned to be what she calls "a good patient," but the book itself refuses this posture: she offers no false resurrections of the spirit. She insists on the tyranny of the body and its damage. Her situation was an extreme one, but it gave form and justification to how I was living then, silently: my own existence defined by injury.

Most of the negative Amazon reviews of *Autobiography of a Face* focus on the idea of self-pity: "She was a sad woman who never got beyond her own personal pain," "I found this book extremely sorrowful and drowning in self-pity," "it seems like she could only think of herself, her complete misery and pain at being 'ugly.'"

A man named "Tom" writes:

> In all of the books I've read, I've never encountered such terribly [sic] moaning and wallowing in self-pity. I can easily sum up the entire 240-page book in 3 words: Woe is me . . . In addition to a mess of crying, the author cannot seem to make up her mind on anything. First she says she does not want to be felt sorry for by anyone, then she proceeds to scorn others about their inability to feel an ounce of sympathy.

The woman Tom describes, "wallowing" in self-pity and unable to decide what the world should do about it, is exactly the woman I grew up afraid of becoming. I knew better—we all, it seems, knew better—than to become one of *those* women who plays victim, lurks around the sickbed, hands her pain out like a business card. What I'm trying to say is, I don't think this was just me. An entire generation, the next wave, grew up doing everything we could to avoid this identity: we take refuge in self-awareness, self-deprecation, jadedness, sarcasm. The Girl Who Cried Pain: she doesn't need meds; she needs a sedative.

And now we find ourselves torn. We don't want anyone to feel sorry for us, but we miss the sympathy when it doesn't come. Feeling sorry for ourselves has become a secret crime—a kind of shameful masturbation—that would chase away the sympathy of others if we ever let it show. "Because I had grown up denying myself any feeling that even hinted at self-pity," Grealy writes, "I now had to find a way to reshape it."

Reshape it into what? Into faith, sexual promiscuity, intellectual ambition. At the pinnacle: into art. Grealy offers this last alchemy, pain-to-art, as possibility but not redemption. It seems likely that for all her wound has given her—perspective, the grit of survival, an insightful meditation on beauty—Grealy would still trade back these wound boons for a pretty face. This confession of willingness is her greatest gift of honesty, not arguing that beauty was more important than profundity, just admitting that she might have chosen it—that beauty was more difficult to live without.

Interlude: Outward

When I started writing this essay, I decided to crowdsource. I wrote a message to some of my favorite women asking them to tell me about their thoughts on female pain. "Please don't not-respond," I wrote; "it would make me feel totally alone in my obsession with gendered woundedness." They responded.

"Perhaps too obvious," wrote a friend in divinity school, "but the fall?" She pointed out that Eve is defined by the pain of childbirth. Another friend suggested that perhaps childbirth shapes women as a horizon of anticipation. Women come into consciousness, she speculated, imagining a future pain toward which their bodies inevitably propel them.

A friend described an upbringing "thoroughly, thoroughly obsessed with not being a victim." She typed *not being a victim* in italics. Another friend described her young devotion to the oeuvre of Lurlene McDaniel, an author who writes about sick girls—cancer-ridden, heart-transplanted, bulimic—who make friends with even sicker girls, girls turned angelic by illness, and always eventually watch these sicker girls die. These books offered an opportunity for two-pronged empathy—the chance to identify with martyr and survivor, to die and live at once, to feel simultaneously the glory of tragedy and the reassurance of continuance.

I got confessions. One friend admitted that female pain often felt, to her, like "a failure of an ethic of care," and that her ideal of feminine pain might be the grieving Madonna: "the pain of care whose object of care has been removed." She was afraid this ideal made her a secret misogynist. Another friend—Taryn, a poet—confessed that her greatest fear was that her poems would come across as solipsistic transcriptions of private suffering, and that in this self-concern they would also register as somehow "feminine." She too was afraid that this first fear made her a secret misogynist.

One friend got so worked up by my e-mail that she waited until the next morning to reply. She was tired of an abiding societal fascination, she wrote, with women who identified themselves by their pain—women who hurt themselves, or got too drunk, or slept with the wrong men. She was more than *tired of.* She was angry.

I think her anger is asking a question, and I think that question demands an answer. How do we represent female pain without producing a culture in which this pain has been fetishized to the point of fantasy or imperative? *Fetishize:* to be excessively or irrationally devoted to. Here is the danger of wounded womanhood: that its invocation will corroborate a pain cult that keeps legitimating, almost legislating, more of itself.

The hard part is that underneath this obscene fascination with women who hurt themselves and have bad sex and drink too much, there are actual women who hurt themselves and have bad sex and drink too much. Female pain is prior to its representation, even if its manifestations are shaped and bent by cultural models.

Relying too much on the image of the wounded woman is reductive, but so is rejecting it—being unwilling to look at the varieties of need and suffering that yield it. We don't want to *be* wounds ("No, you're the wound!") but we should be allowed to have them, to speak about having them, to be something more than just another girl who has one. We should be able to do these things without failing the feminism of our mothers, and we should be able to represent women who hurt without walking backward into a voyeuristic rehashing of the old cultural models: another emo cutter under the bleachers, another hurt-seeking missile of womanhood, a body gone drunk or bruised or barren, another archetype sunk into blackout under the sheets.

We've got a Janus-faced relationship to female pain. We're attracted to it and revolted by it; proud and ashamed of it. So we've developed a post-wounded voice, a stance of numbness or crutch of sarcasm that implies pain without claiming it, that seems to stave off certain accusations it can see on the horizon: melodrama, triviality, wallowing—an ethical and aesthetic commandment: Don't valorize suffering women.

You court a certain disdain by choosing to write about hurting women. You get your period with sharks around—*exposed column of nerve and blood*—but everyone thinks it's a stupid show. You want to cry, *I am not a melodramatic person!* But everyone thinks you are. You're willing to bleed but it looks, instead, like you're trying to get bloody. When you bleed like that—all over everything, tempting the sharks—you get told you're corroborating the wrong mythology. You should be ashamed of yourself. *Plug it up.*

In 1844, a woman named Harriet Martineau wrote a book called *Life in the Sick Room.* Ten years later, she published an autobiography. In this second book, she compresses her illness to a footnote, explaining: "There is no point of which I am more sure than it is unwise in sick people to keep a diary." She knew better than to yoke her identity as an author to her status as a sick woman, especially in a culture eager to see women as invalids-in-waiting. Perhaps she was justifiably afraid that her sickness would be understood as limiting the scope of her vision, that it might quarantine her into category. *A major poet with a minor range:* The Passion of the Invalid.

Lucy Grealy learned to be a good patient when she learned that it was possible to fail at being sick. "My feelings of shame and guilt for failing not to suffer," she writes, "became more unbearable. The physical pain seemed almost easy in comparison." Sometimes we call *failing not to suffer* something else: we call it wallowing. Wallow, intr. v.: to roll the body about indolently or clumsily, as if in snow, water, or mud; to luxuriate, to revel. This is the fear: that we will turn our bodies clumsy if we spend too much time mourning what has happened to them; if we revel in our pain like a shark-infested sea; if we wear the mud like paint across our skin-stripped bodies.

Wound #13

When Misfit Molly was twenty-four, a stranger broke into her Brooklyn apartment and tried to rape her at knifepoint. She was able to get away—fleeing her studio naked, after a ten-minute struggle—but of course that didn't release her from years of fear, years of trying to make sense of what had happened. "Imposing a truly sensible narrative on my attack," she writes, "proved impossible in its aftermath." She moved in with a good friend, and they watched films to help them fall asleep at night:

> We turned to what we wanted to watch, and that happened, reflexively, to be stories about women in peril, women without autonomy, girls who disappear, dark ladies hurting within and without. On the subway, I found myself obsessively listening to old-time murder ballads like "Pretty Polly," fascinated by the perverse beauty of lyrics like "He stabbed her through the heart and her heart's blood did flow."

Dark ladies hurting within and without. It doesn't surprise me that Molly was drawn to them. Maybe they gave her visions of pain worse than her own, or made her feel less alone, or simply granted her permission to inhabit her own pain by offering a world in which the logic of pain held court.

This essay isn't fighting for that world. It isn't simply criticizing the post-wounded voice, or dismissing the ways in which female pain gets dismissed. I do believe there is nothing shameful about being in pain, and I do mean for this essay to be a manifesto against the accusation of wallowing. But the essay isn't a double negative, a dismissal of dismissal, so much as a search for possibility—the possibility of representing female suffering without reifying its mythos.

Lucy Grealy describes much of her artistic life as an attempt "to grant myself the complicated and necessary right to suffer."

I'm looking for the thirteenth nude, who arrives at the close of Carson's poem:

> Very much like Nude #1.
> And yet utterly different.
> . . .
> I saw it was a human body
>
> trying to stand against winds so terrible that the flesh was
>   blowing off the bones.
> And there was no pain.
> The wind
>
> was cleansing the bones.
> They stood forth silver and necessary.
> It was not my body, not a woman's body, it was the body of us all.
> It walked out of the light.

This Nude is like the first Nude because she is nothing but ragged flesh, but here the "flesh [is] blowing off" and her nakedness signals strength. Her exposure is clean and necessary. There is no pain. The nerves are gone. The move away from pain requires a movement into commonality: "out of the light" of human particularity and gender ("It was not my body, not a woman's body") and into the Universal ("it was the body of us all"). Walking out of the light simultaneously suggests being constituted by this light—walking forth from the substance of origin—and leaving it behind, abandoning the state of visible representation. Once pain is cleansed into something silver and necessary, it no longer needs to be illuminated. Pain only reaches beyond itself when its damage shifts from private to public, from solipsistic to collective.

One friend sent me a letter about pain, written on a piece of nearly translucent paper. She suggested we could see our wounds as "places of conductivity where the pain hits your experience and lights something up." Her translucent paper mattered. I could see the world beyond her words: the table, my own fingers. Perhaps this visibility—this invitation to see parts in relation—is what pain makes possible.

We shouldn't forget how this thirteenth Nude recalls the first one, that primal artifact of pain, whose bloody ghost limns these silver bones like an aura, reminding us that the cleansing cannot happen without some loss: *cleaned out the rot, left me mouthfull of love.* Like Stevens and his thirteen blackbirds, we see pain from every angle; no single posture of suffering is allowed any measure of perceptual tyranny. We can't see suffering one way; we have to look at it from thirteen directions and that is only the beginning—then we are called to follow this figure striding out of the light.

We follow this figure into contradiction, into a confession that wounds are desired and despised; that they grant power and come at a price; that suffering yields virtue and selfishness; that victimhood is a mix of situation and agency; that pain is the object of representation and also its product; that culture transcribes genuine suffering while naturalizing its symptoms. We follow this thirteenth nude back to the bleachers, where some girl is putting on a Passion Play with her razor. We should watch. She's hurting, but that doesn't mean she'll hurt forever—or that hurt is the only identity she can own. There is a way of representing female consciousness that can witness pain but also witness a larger self around that pain—a self who grows larger than its scars without disowning them, who is neither wound-dwelling nor jaded, who is actually healing.

We can watch what happens when the girl under the bleachers puts down the blade. Suffering is interesting but so is getting better. The aftermath of wounds—the strain and struggle of stitching the skin, the stride of silver bones—contours women alongside the wounds themselves. Glück dreams of "a harp, its string cutting / deep into my palm. In the dream, / it both makes the wound and seals the wound."

When I read Taryn's poems, I see imagination twining like a vine out of injury. You can see bits of her life—a major surgery to remove a tumor wrapped around her liver—but the prone body of her female subject ("she is laid out supplicant") is never the only body in view. This female voice is never allowed any monopoly on hurt. The poems are thick with damage—a gardener's birds with their thin bones snapped, a dead fat doe ("Her delicious odor!")—and butchering instructions: "Spread the ribs with a stick . . . accordion of bone glows beneath. Reveal the leg meat. This is like opening a set of French doors." These verbs are verbs of opening, slicing, parting, exploring, excavating, and extracting. Damage isn't for its own sake. It's for epistemology or else it's for dinner. *Sometimes you're nothing but meat, girl.* Where others might navel-gaze, Taryn is opening the navels of animals—*not my body, not a woman's body*—but her gaze feels personal in its vulnerability. She offers a sense of the violence intrinsic to the feat of living in a body—any body, among other bodies—an awareness necessarily embedded in the body of us all, that body made of light and departing from it.

I want to honor what happens when confession collides with butchering instructions: how we find an admission of wounds but also a vision of manipulating bloody bodies, arranging and opening their parts. I want to insist that female pain is still news. It's always news. We've never already heard it.

It's news when a girl loses her virginity or gets an ache in the rag and bone shop of her heart. It's news when she starts getting her period or when she does something to make herself stop. It's news if a woman feels terrible about herself in the world—anywhere, anytime, ever. It's news whenever a girl has an abortion because her abortion has never been had before and won't ever be had again. I'm saying this as someone who's had an abortion but hasn't had anyone else's.

Sure, some news is bigger news than other news. War is bigger news than a girl having mixed feelings about the way some guy fucked her and didn't call. But I don't believe in a finite economy of empathy; I happen to think that paying attention yields as much as it taxes. You learn to start seeing.

I think dismissing female pain as overly familiar or somehow out-of-date—twice-told, thrice-told, 1,001-nights-told—masks deeper accusations: that suffering women are playing victim, going weak, or choosing self-indulgence over bravery. I think dismissing wounds offers a convenient excuse: no need to struggle with the listening or telling anymore. *Plug it up.* Like somehow our task is to inhabit the jaded aftermath of terminal self-awareness once the story of all pain has already been told.

For a long time I have hesitated to write a book on woman, is how de Beauvoir starts one of the most famous books on women ever written. *The subject is irritating, especially to women; and it is not new.* Sometimes I feel like I'm beating a dead wound. But I say: keep bleeding. Just write toward something beyond blood.

The wounded woman gets called a stereotype and sometimes she is. But sometimes she's just true. I think the possibility of fetishizing pain is no reason to stop representing it. Pain that gets performed is still pain. Pain turned trite is still pain. I think the charges of cliché and performance offer our closed hearts too many alibis, and I want our hearts to be open. I just wrote that. I want our hearts to be open. I mean it.

Works Consulted

Books

Agee, James, and Walker Evans. *Let Us Now Praise Famous Men.*

Baxter, Charles. *Burning Down the House: Essays on Fiction.*

Bidart, Frank. "Ellen West," in *The Book of the Body.*

Brooks, Peter. *Troubling Confessions: Speaking Guilt in Law and Literature.*

Capote, Truman. *In Cold Blood.*

Carson, Anne. "The Glass Essay" and "Teresa of God," in *Glass, Irony and God.*

D'Ambrosio, Charles. *Orphans.*

De Beauvoir, Simone. *The Second Sex.*

Dickens, Charles. *David Copperfield.*

———. *Great Expectations.*

Didion, Joan. *Salvador.*

———. *Slouching Towards Bethlehem.*

———. *The White Album.*

Dubus, Andre. *Meditations from a Movable Chair.*

Flaubert, Gustave. *Madame Bovary.*

Grealy, Lucy. *Autobiography of a Face.*

Hass, Robert. "Images," in *Twentieth Century Pleasures.*

Hemingway, Ernest. *For Whom the Bell Tolls.*

Heti, Sheila. *How Should a Person Be?*

Huggan, Graham. *The Postcolonial Exotic: Marketing the Margins.*

Huxley, Thomas, *Man's Place in Nature.*

Kahlo, Frida. *Diary.*

Keen, Suzanne. *Empathy and the Novel.*

Knapp, Caroline. *Drinking: A Love Story.*

———. *Appetites: Why Women Want.*

Kundera, Milan. *The Unbearable Lightness of Being.*

Malcolm, Janet. *The Journalist and the Murderer.*

Manguso, Sarah. *The Two Kinds of Decay.*

Martineau, Harriet. *Autobiography.*

Merleau-Ponty, Maurice. *Phenomenology of Perception.*

Nussbaum, Martha C. *Cultivating Humanity: A Classical Defense of Reform in Liberal Education.*

———. *Poetic Justice: The Literary Imagination and Public Life.*

Plath, Sylvia. "Cut," "Ariel," "Daddy," in *Ariel.*

Pope, Alexander. *The Rape of the Lock.*

Propp, Vladimir. *Morphology of the Folktale.*

Scarry, Elaine. *The Body in Pain: The Making and Unmaking of the World.*

Schwilling, Taryn. *The Anatomist.*

Smith, Adam. *Theory of Moral Sentiments.*

Solomon, Robert. *In Defense of Sentimentality.*

Sontag, Susan. *Illness as Metaphor.*

———. *Regarding the Pain of Others.*

Stevens, Wallace. *The Necessary Angel.*

———. "The Revolutionists Stop for Orangeade" and "The Motive for Metaphor," in *The Palm at the End of the Mind.*

Stoker, Bram. *Dracula.*

Tolstoy, Leo. *Anna Karenina.*

Vollmann, William T. *Poor People.*

Wallace, David Foster. *Infinite Jest.*

Wilde, Oscar. *De Profundis.*

Yeats, William Butler. "The Circus Animals' Desertion," in *Last Poems.*

Žižek, Slavoj. *First As Tragedy, Then As Farce.*

Essays, Articles, and Stories

Barthelme, Donald. "Wrack." *New Yorker,* October 21, 1972: 36–37.

Boyle, Molly. "How Murder Ballads Helped." *Hairpin,* April 19, 2012.
http://thehairpin.com/2012/04/how-murder-ballads-helped-me.

Browne, Sir Thomas. "Letter to a Friend."

Decety, Jean. "The Neurodevelopment of Empathy in Humans."
Developmental Neuroscience 32:4 (2010): 257–267.

Gawande, Atul. "The Itch." *New Yorker,* June 30, 2008: 58–65.

Hoffmann, Diane E., and Anita J. Tarzian. "The Girl Who Cried Pain:
A Bias Against Women in the Treatment of Pain." *Journal of Law,
Medicine & Ethics* 29:1 (Spring 2001): 13–27.

Hungerford, Amy. "Cold Fiction." *Yale Review* 99:1 (January 2011).

Irving, John. "In Defense of Sentimentality." *New York Times,*
November 25, 1979.

Jefferson, Mark. "What Is Wrong with Sentimentality?" *Mind* 92 (1983):
519–529.

Johnson, John A., Jonathan M. Cheek, and Robert Smither. "The
Structure of Empathy." *Journal of Personality and Social Psychology*
45:6 (1983): 1299–1312.

Morens, David. "At the Deathbed of Consumptive Art." *Emerging Infectious
Diseases* 8:11 (2002): 1353–1358.

Robbins, Michael. "The Constant Gardener: On Louise Glück." *Los Angeles
Review of Books,* December 4, 2012.

Rorty, Richard. "Human Rights, Rationality, and Sentimentality," in
On Human Rights: The Oxford Amnesty Lectures, ed. Stephen Shute
and Susan Hurley. New York: Basic Books, 1993.

Tanner, Michael. "Sentimentality." *Proceedings of the Aristotelian Society* 77
(1976–77): 127–147.

Tompkins, Jane. "Sentimental Power: *Uncle Tom's Cabin* and the Politics
of Literary History," in *Sensational Designs: The Cultural Work of
American Fiction, 1790–1860,* 122–146. New York: Oxford University
Press, 1985.

Wallace, David Foster. "The Empty Plenum: David Markson's *Wittgenstein's
Mistress.*" *Review of Contemporary Fiction* 10:2 (Summer 1990).

Wood, James. "Tides of Treacle." *London Review of Books* 27:12 (June 23, 2005).

Zahavi, Dan, and Soren Overgaard. "Empathy Without Isomorphism: A Phenomenological Account," in *Empathy: From Bench to Bedside.* Cambridge, MA: MIT Press, 2012.

Musical and Dramatic Works

Amos, Tori. "Blood Roses," "Jackie's Strength," "Silent All These Years."

Björk. "Bachelorette."

Bush, Kate. "Experiment IV," "Wuthering Heights."

DiFranco, Ani. "Buildings and Bridges," "Independence Day," "Pixie," "Pulse," "Swan Dive."

Guns N' Roses. "Sentimental Movie."

Lewis, Leona. "Bleeding Love."

Puccini, Giacomo. *La Bohème.*

Verdi, Guiseppe. *La Traviata.*

Williams, Tennessee. *A Streetcar Named Desire.*

Carrie, dir. Brian De Palma. 1976.

Girls, created by Lena Dunham. 2012–13.

Paradise Lost: The Child Murders at Robin Hood Hills (1996), *Paradise Lost 2: Revelations* (2000), *Paradise Lost 3: Purgatory* (2011). Dir. Joe Berlinger and Bruce Sinofsky.

Women consulted for "Grand Unified Theory of Female Pain"

Molly Boyle, Lily Brown, Casey Cep, Harriet Clark, Merve Emre, Rachel Fagnant, Miranda Featherstone, Michelle Huneven, Colleen Kinder, Emily Matchar, Kyle McCarthy, Katie Parry, Kiki Petrosino, Nadya Pittendregh, Jaime Powers, Taryn Schwilling, Aria Sloss, Bridget Talone, Moira Weigel, and Jenny Zhang.

Acknowledgments

I'm grateful to the journals where these essays first appeared: "The Empathy Exams," "Immortal Horizon," and "The Broken Heart of James Agee" in the *Believer* ("The Broken Heart of James Agee" reprinted in *American Writers on Class*); "Devil's Bait" in *Harper's* (reprinted in *The Best American Essays 2014*); "Fog Count" in *Oxford American*; "Grand Unified Theory of Female Pain" in the *Virginia Quarterly Review*; "Morphology of the Hit," "La Plata Perdida," "Lost Boys," and "Sublime, Revised" in *A Public Space*; "La Frontera" in *VICE*; "Indigenous to the Hood" in *Los Angeles Review of Books*; "Ex-Votos" and "Servicio Supercompleto" in the *Paris Review Daily* (reprinted in *Paper Darts*); "In Defense of Saccharin(e)" in *Black Warrior Review*.

It was an honor to work with many wonderful editors along the way: Rocco Castoro, Wes Enzinna, Deirdre Foley-Mendelssohn, Olivia Harrington, Roger Hodge, Heidi Julavits, Daniel Levin Becker, James Marcus, Anne McPeak, Andi Mudd, Colin Rafferty, Shelly Reed, Matthew Specktor, Karolina Waclawiak, Allison Wright, and of course Brigid Hughes at *A Public Space*—who has believed in my work since the very beginning. Much gratitude to Max Porter at Granta UK, who has promised the title tattooed in Gill Sans across his back.

Thanks also to my advisors at Yale—Amy Hungerford, Wai Chee Dimock, and Caleb Smith—who have been helpful and gracious as I've balanced my critical and creative lives. I feel an abiding and evolving gratitude to Charlie D'Ambrosio, who taught me early that the problem with an essay can eventually become its subject.

I am lucky to have an incredible agent in Jin Auh, tireless and fearsome champion, and I am genuinely blessed she helped this book find a home at Graywolf. Thank you Katie Dublinski, Erin Kottke, Fiona McCrae, Michael Taeckens, Steve Woodward, and especially Jeff Shotts, who has been a soulmate and stalwart from the first moment he laid his green pen on this manuscript.

I feel gratitude for the friendship, support, and guidance of so many people, especially Aria Sloss, Colleen Kinder, Harriet Clark, Rachel Fagnant, Kyle McCarthy, and Nam Le; Rebecaa Buckwalter-Poza, Chelsea Catalanotto, Casey Cep, Alexis Chema, Liz Cunningham, Charlotte Douglas, Merve Emre, Miranda Featherstone, Micah Fitzerman-Blue, Norm, Amy, Andrew, and Will Gorin, Michelle Huneven, Margot Kaminski, Elyssa Kilman, Lindsay Levine, Jess Marsh, Emily Matchar, Amalia McGibbon, Tara Menon, Cat Moore, Max Nicholas, Ben Nugent, Katie Parry, Jen Percy, Eve Peters, Kiki Petrosino, Caitlin Pilla, Nadya Pittendrigh, Jamie Powers, Amber Qureshi, Jeremy Reff, Liba Rubenstein, Jake Rubin, Taryn Schwilling, Sabrina Serrantino, Nina Siegal, Mary Simmons, Aria Sloss, Meg Swertlow, Susan Szmyt, Robin Wasserman, Julia Whicker, Abby Wild, and Jenny Zhang.

To Dave, finally, thank you: This book wouldn't be, without you.

I'm grateful to my entire family—tangled and wonderful—and in particular to my courageous and compassionate mother, Joanne, to whom this book is dedicated with admiration and love.

Judge's Afterword

Masters in the art of thinking against oneself, Nietzsche,
Baudelaire, and Dostoevsky have taught us to side with our
dangers, to broaden the sphere of our diseases, to acquire
existence by division from our being.

—E. M. CIORAN

The fate of our insights is often perilous, as though even our most elementary thinking were a resistant signal only transmittable through static, or disappearing ink. Many have sought to operate along the borders of the body, pain, shame, defiance, vision, and doubt without double-crossing those insights with ready-made glamour, whether charm or scorn. Near the conclusion of her own magnificent 1994 reconnaissance of those elusive psychic perimeters, *Autobiography of a Face*, Lucy Grealy wrote:

> I used to think truth was eternal, that once I *knew*, once I *saw*, it would be with me forever, a constant by which everything else could be measured. I know now that this isn't so, that most truths are inherently unretainable, that we have to work all our lives to remember the most basic things.

Grealy is one of the provisional guides Leslie Jamison invokes in *The Empathy Exams*, along with Caroline Knapp, James Agee, Frida Kahlo, Joan Didion, Anne Carson, Susan Sontag, Elaine Scarry, and Vladimir Propp, among others, and something of Grealy's canniness and persistence spurs Jamison. As readers (maybe also authors) we are so acclimated to reductive and tidy literary niches, enclosures, and genres—can the book in our hands safely be branded a memoir, a collection of essays, reportage, science, anthropology, cultural criticism, theory?—that when we chance upon a work and a writer who summons and dares the full tilt of all her volatile resources, intellectual and emotional, personal and historical, the effect is, well, disorienting, astonishing. "We crash into wonder," as she says, and the span of topics Jamison tosses up is correspondingly smashing and wondrous: medical actors, sentimentality, violence, plastic surgery, guilt, diseases, the Barkley Marathons, stylish "ex-votos" for exemplary artists, incarceration, wounds, scars, fear, yearning, community, and the mutations of physical pain.

Veering from anatomy into argument, thinking itself—articulation, representation—proves the provocation and ultimate subject of *The Empathy Exams*. "I had to write these essays," she recounts, "to discover the questions they were asking."

Decades ago, for another context, E. M. Cioran once dubbed Jamison's rare and beautiful mode "thinking against oneself," and her formal embodiments of her self-suspicion are as dazzling as tough-minded—her casually bravura recital of a random street attack via Propp's *Morphology of the Folktale*, the infinite regressions of her medical acting, where "Leslie Jamison" is another case study, the collage and crowdsourcing of her "Grand Unified Theory of Female Pain," and the contrapuntal staccato inside her lyricism. "I kept running into an opacity at the core of bodily experience," she says, "a resistance to language, an empty center: how can pain *mean*? . . . The essays in this book were memoir until they couldn't stand to be memoir anymore."

Robert Polito

May 2013

Confession and Community

This essay by Leslie Jamison originally appeared in The Guardian *and is reprinted here with permission.*

Confessional writing often gets a bad rap. People call it self-absorbed, solipsistic, self-indulgent. Who wants to hear another thirty-year-old going on and on about her damage? But when I published a collection of "confessional" essays this spring, *The Empathy Exams,* full of personal material (an abortion, heart surgery, getting punched in the face by a stranger)— I started to feel like confession could be the opposite of solipsism. My confessions elicited responses. They coaxed chorus like a brushfire.

After my book came out, I found myself becoming an unwitting confessor to countless strangers: I heard from a woman with chronic headaches, a man struggling with the aftermath of being circumcised at eighteen, a woman dealing with the death of her pet chicken, a high-school senior trying to process her best friend's eating disorder, a homeless substitute teacher in Minneapolis, a neurologist trying to stay on the career track after multiple medical leaves of absence. I heard from doctors who'd given the book to their medical students; medical students who'd given it to their professors. I heard from a preacher who'd used it in his Good Friday sermon.

I loved seeing the way my words traveled beyond the pages and became about so much more than what I'd lived, or what I'd felt. My writing was like a grown up child suddenly taking up residence in all sorts of strange places and sending back photos.

There are many ways to confess and many ways confession can reach beyond itself. If the definition of solipsism is "a theory holding that the self can know nothing but its own modifications and that the self is the only existent thing," then little pushes back against solipsism more forcefully than confession gone public. This kind of confession inevitably creates dialogue.

I've felt this as a reader as well, encountering confessional narratives whose revelations felt more like forking paths than private cloisters: Eula Biss's *Notes from No Man's Land* shares private moments of bodily experience—collisions, exhaustion, sensory wonder—in a way that feels deeply committed to exploring what it means to be part of a collective public body, fraught with issues of race and class and guilt; and Rebecca Solnit's *The Faraway Nearby* places a deeply personal narrative—reckoning with her mother's dementia, with the longer arc of their tumultuous relationship—inside a broader constellation of stories, Inuit myths, scientific inquiries, tales of heroes, and monsters and ice.

When I read each of these deeply personal books, I didn't feel as if it was the product of a self that didn't know anything beyond itself—I felt as if it was the product of a self that somehow, miraculously, knew me as well, or at least knew about things that included me.

I first read Lucy Grealy's *Autobiography of a Face*—a memoir about her childhood illness and subsequent disfigurement—when I was recovering from major jaw surgery, and I felt the urge to shout "Amen!" on nearly every page. Her willingness to linger inside trauma—to excavate more meaning rather than yielding to the sense that she had dwelled too long—felt less like self-involvement and more like a gift. I didn't feel excluded; I felt my whole life summoned into the narrative. And as an author, in turn, I was summoned into the lives of those who had read me.

Confession doesn't just allow—it incites. Someone tweeted about my essays: "After reading this book, I want to write about my hidden pain until my fingers bleed, and then I want to write about my bleeding fingers." One woman wrote to me to say that as she was writing, her mother was collecting her things from her ex-boyfriend's house: "I don't know how to hold this hurt inside," she said. "But I'm mortified at the thought of talking about it or writing about it or painting it—somehow that seems so much more embarrassing than drunk-dialing him, or falling off a bar stool and breaking my wrist, or whatever ways used to seem like options."

Another woman wrote to say that one of my essays had made her turn down sex with a guy who didn't love her. "As low as that sounds," she said, as if it didn't matter much. But it mattered to me. It didn't sound low at all. It sounded like something I might have needed—at several points in my life—to hear. She told me she was writing drunk. She'd needed to get drunk to find the courage to write at all.

As I got more notes from strangers, I started to wonder what desires motivated them. What do readers want from the writers they read? What sorts of responses do they imagine? Sometimes a reader offers his own life;

sometimes he only offers praise. Every offering suggests itself as a mixture of gift and request—a desire to show the author what her words have meant, and a desire to be seen: "Let me know I'm visible to you, as you've been visible to me."

When I published fiction, I'd also receive notes from strangers—a real estate agent in Hawaii who said my short story gave him a better understanding of why his younger sister slept with so many men, a rowdy frat boy who said my writing inspired him to treat women better. A few years after my first novel was published, I got an email from a woman who'd read it and hated it and regretted spending a dime on it in a thrift store. (She swore to this; it had only cost ten cents.) She said it had made her lose all hope of staying sober. She said I should be ashamed of sending that much hopelessness into the world. She said she'd put a lot of drugs into her body that morning. She said she hoped she didn't last through the day. Her resentment and disappointment held such clear notes of yearning—the hunger for deliverance, the hope that a novel or an essay or a single sentence might offer it. I could understand this impulse to get in touch: if it felt like an author had already come into your life, already seen some aspect of your experience then it would be natural to want to extend this intimacy into conversation.

The impulse to contact a confessional writer—whose writing has already revealed something private—is something else. Perhaps it is still a desire to translate one kind of intimacy into another, but the terms are different. With confessional writing, the disclosure has already happened—now the reader wants to confess something back, make a reciprocal exchange. So whenever people talk about confessional writing as navel-gazing or self-involved, I think about those voices, and their offerings.

When they confessed things to me, these strangers were offering something but they were also asking for something. They were asking for the subject of the book itself: empathy. They wanted an enactment of its central principle, its primary call: to pay attention. Even when they didn't say they wanted this, I felt I owed it to them. The professor struggling with chronic headaches wasn't asking for anything, she was just offering a response: "I find the thing that wears you down the most is pain. To wake up and as you gain consciousness to feel the pain again, and wanting it to not be so, but yet it is, and having to face that reality hundreds, in my case thousands, of days in a row. It transforms you and disconnects you from everyone, even those who want to understand."

Notes from strangers were gifts and burdens at once. They made me think about what I'd written near the end of my collection: "I don't believe in a finite economy of empathy." Someone on Instagram had even turned this into a hashtag: #idontbelieveinafiniteeconomyofempathy. But, I started to wonder, was it true?

An artist from Los Angeles sent a note about how strange he felt about sending a note: "So many of your readers will feel exactly this way, and think, 'Wow, I feel the same things too! We should be friends, like for real!' . . . imagine that they can suspend the adult world and just reach, shoulder against the screen, an arm into the computer and have it somehow emerge out of your screen, into your life, in a manner that is not reaching or grasping, but rather extending and giving, not freakish and bizarre, but surprising and wonderful. At best, even a welcoming, non-flailing arm, coming from out of your screen, waving hello, or offering a pistachio, or book, will still seem, at best, unnatural."

He was right: there were arms coming out of my screen, asking for something even when they weren't. There were too many of them. I couldn't respond to all of them. At a certain point I stopped responding to any of them. I didn't respond to the one who wrote to me drunk, the one who wrote to me after her relationship had ended, to the man in the shelter or the man in the retirement home. An abiding sense of guilt and hypocrisy began to fester: I was peddling empathy everywhere, and getting so much from it—absorbing the affirmation of every charged emotional response to what I'd written. I'd made everyone feel, and now I was ignoring those feelings. I was empathetic in the abstract and stingy everywhere else.

Every stop on the book tour pushed me up against the limits of myself, forced me to confront the finitude of the economy I'd once called infinite. Every city offered questions that felt full of invisible emotional baggage: Washington, DC, was a woman getting irritated about the notion that faking empathy could ever do anyone any good. SoHo, in New York, was a girl with the seismograph of an electrocardiogram tattooed across her chest. San Francisco was a friend hopping up the stairs on crutches, a doctor saying she wanted more room for her heart in the medicine she practiced. Kalamazoo was homemade chocolate-covered pretzels and a woman with chronic lupus. The city of Ann Arbor was a girl in black eyeliner and high-top sneakers telling me that she'd never believed her stories were worth telling, all those drunken nights and regrets, but that now she thought her life might be worth narrating after all.

Through all this, I was gathering signatures and messages in a tour copy of the book. This was my attempt at reciprocity: whenever someone asked me to sign her book, I would ask her to sign mine. It was a way to create, for a moment, the kind of symmetry that felt impossible in the letters I received. Someone wrote: "Your words have opened me, flayed me, improved me." Someone else: "It's so nice to meet another 'wound-dweller.'" Another: "I'm sorry I laughed during the soul-nailed-to-the-cross part of the reading." Next to a section headed "OB GYN" (for obstetrics and gynecology), one woman wrote: "Just went yesterday! Scaling menopause mountain." And next to a section about my experience with supraventricular tachycardia, another wrote: "SVT is the fucking worst." Or: "We are kindred spirits." Or: "This gave me solace." Or: "I carry your heart."

I remember looking into the eyes of a woman in Kalamazoo—who had been ill for years with chronic fatigue—and she was telling me about her illness, but the whole time she was talking I was picturing the bath tub in the old wooden B&B where I was staying. I was picturing that bathtub, or wondering if I was confusing it with the bathroom in the university guest house by the river in Iowa City, or the glass-walled shrine in my sleek modern hotel in Minneapolis. This woman was telling me it felt like there wouldn't ever be an end to how she hurt—and I knew the truth, which is that for me there would be: the ending had taken the shape of a bathtub in my mind.

Readings also held moments of doubt and resistance. One night in Boise, Idaho, after I'd finished reading an essay about James Agee—how I'd read his account of sharecropper families one autumn, after being punched in the face in Nicaragua, and how his guilt had resonated with the guilt I felt about visiting a country whose poverty I'd never faced myself. I'd written about a little boy named Luis, who'd slept one night outside the house where I was staying, and how I hadn't invited him to sleep inside, and how guilty I'd felt—and how that guilt had made me feel closer to Agee, closer to his overblown version of self-doubt and anguish. I was pretty sure I'd spun my own guilt into something beautiful. I often read the essay out loud because I felt proud of the cadences in its closing paragraph. After I was done, a boy stood up and asked: "Why didn't you let that boy into the house?" I felt like saying: that's what the whole essay is about. But his question seemed to be suggesting that my self-awareness hadn't answered the question: it hadn't dissolved any problems, only illuminated them more fully.

What lies behind this feeling of being owed something by the authors we read? It was the sense of being called on for instructions—for hope, for a plan—that started to feel daunting; its futility no longer catalyzing (my words can change something) so much as dispiriting (but they can't change much). Increasingly, I found myself called on to offer some kind of blueprint for what empathy itself might look like. I did a radio show with a famous psychologist who talked about his decades of research while I talked about my feelings, or thoughts I'd had in the shower. It felt false to be labeled an empathy expert. I felt more like a salesman. I felt distinctly unqualified.

There was a particular hypocrisy that attached to the fact that it was always empathy I was talking about. Empathy is all about otherness, but my relationship to empathy was largely about me—my book, my career. I usually passed the homeless man who stood near my subway stop without giving him anything, because I was always in a rush: heading to the airport, or a photo shoot, or some radio studio downtown; I needed to get somewhere and talk to someone about caring for everyone. At Newark airport, in New Jersey, snapping a photo of my book I'd found in the airport bookstore, I kept backing up to get a better crop and I nearly knocked over a woman with a cane. What would I have said? Excuse me while I injure you, I'm just trying to get a better angle on my empathy book vanity shot.

The unanswered notes in my inbox stopped feeling like affirmation and started feeling like proof of a certain abiding hypocrisy: all the people I wasn't engaging with as I went around singing the praises of engagement.

"Kitsch causes two tears to flow in quick succession," Milan Kundera writes. "The first tear says: how nice to see children running on the grass! The second tear says: How nice to be moved, together with all mankind, by children running on the grass!" We love to feel ourselves loving strangers—or, at the very least, considering the ways we might love them more. But in the end, it's not about the stars in my inbox, reminding me to respond, or even my guilt about those stars, or my guilt about the money I didn't give, or the advice I couldn't offer. It's about the people who looked me in the eye—in Ann Arbor, San Francisco, Kalamazoo—and said: this gave me permission to talk about what hurt. To them, I say: thank you for making my confession larger than itself.

The Graywolf Press Nonfiction Prize

The Empathy Exams by Leslie Jamison is the 2011 winner of the Graywolf Press Nonfiction Prize. Graywolf awards this prize every twelve to eighteen months to a previously unpublished, full-length work of outstanding literary nonfiction by a writer who is not yet established in the genre. Previous winners include *The Grey Album: On the Blackness of Blackness* by Kevin Young, *Notes from No Man's Land: American Essays* by Eula Biss, *Black Glasses Like Clark Kent: A GI's Secret from Postwar Japan* by Terese Svoboda, *Neck Deep and Other Predicaments* by Ander Monson, and *Frantic Transmissions to and from Los Angeles: An Accidental Memoir* by Kate Braverman.

The Graywolf Press Nonfiction Prize seeks to acknowledge—and honor—the great traditions of literary nonfiction, extending from Robert Burton and Thomas Browne in the seventeenth century through Daniel Defoe and Lytton Strachey and on to James Baldwin, Joan Didion, and Jamaica Kincaid in our own time. Whether grounded in observation, autobiography, or research, much of the most beautiful, daring, and original writing over the past few decades can be categorized as nonfiction. Graywolf is excited to increase its commitment to the evolving and dynamic genre.

The 2011 prize was judged by Robert Polito, author of *Hollywood & God*, *Savage Art: A Biography of Jim Thompson*, *Doubles*, and *A Reader's Guide to James Merrill's The Changing Light at Sandover*, and formerly director of the graduate writing program at the New School in New York City. He is currently president of the Poetry Foundation in Chicago.

The Graywolf Press Nonfiction Prize is funded in part by endowed gifts from the Arsham Ohanessian Charitable Remainder Unitrust and the Ruth Easton Fund of the Edelstein Family Foundation.

Arsham Ohanessian, an Armenian born in Iraq who came to the United States in 1952, was an avid reader and a tireless advocate for human rights and peace. He strongly believed in the power of literature and education to make a positive impact on humanity.

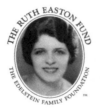

Ruth Easton, born in North Branch, Minnesota, was a Broadway actress in the 1920s and 1930s. The Ruth Easton Fund of the Edelstein Family Foundation is pleased to support the work of emerging artists and writers in her honor.

Graywolf Press is grateful to Arsham Ohanessian and Ruth Easton for their generous support.

LESLIE JAMISON is the author of a novel, *The Gin Closet*, which was a finalist for the *Los Angeles Times* First Fiction Prize. Her essays have appeared in the *Believer*, *Harper's*, *Oxford American*, *A Public Space*, *Tin House*, and *The Best American Essays*. She is a regular columnist for the *New York Times Book Review* and lives in Brooklyn, New York. Find her at www.lesliejamison.com or @lsjamison.

The text of *The Empathy Exams* is set in Adobe Jenson Pro, a typeface drawn by Robert Slimbach and based on late-fifteenth-century types by the printer Nicolas Jenson. This book was designed by Ann Sudmeier. Composition by BookMobile Design & Digital Publisher Services, Minneapolis, Minnesota. Manufactured by Versa Press on acid-free 30 percent postconsumer wastepaper.

Previous Winners of the Graywolf Press Nonfiction Prize

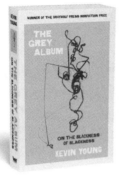

A National Book Critics Circle Award Finalist in Criticism

"An ambitious blast of fact and feeling, a nervy piece of performance art."
—*The New York Times*

Paperback / Ebook available

Winner of the 2010 National Book Critics Circle Award in Criticism

"The most accomplished book of essays anyone has written or published so far in the 21st century."
—*Salon*

Paperback / Ebook available

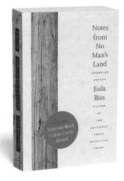

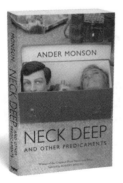

A debut that uses nonliterary forms to delve into a mix of obsessions

"[Monson's] geek act has charm. . . . [He] revels in the way information flows through the world."
—*The New York Times Book Review*

Paperback

 WWW.GRAYWOLFPRESS.ORG

Many Graywolf authors are available to chat with your book club or classroom via phone and Skype. Email us at **wolves@graywolfpress.org** for further details.

Visit **graywolfpress.org** to sign up for our monthly newsletter and to check out our many regularly updated features, including our On Craft series, Pub Talk series, Poem of the Week, author interviews, special sales, book giveaways, tour listings, catalogs, and much more.

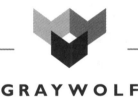

GRAYWOLF
PRESS

Graywolf Press is a leading independent publisher committed to the discovery and energetic publication of contemporary American and international literature. We champion outstanding writers at all stages of their careers to ensure that diverse voices can be heard in a crowded marketplace.

We believe books that nourish the individual spirit and enrich the broader culture must be supported by attentive editing, superior design, and creative promotion.